Nurturing the
Premature Infant

NURTURING THE PREMATURE INFANT

Developmental Interventions in the Neonatal Intensive Care Nursery

Edited by
EDWARD GOLDSON, M.D.

New York   Oxford
OXFORD UNIVERSITY PRESS
1999

Oxford University Press

Oxford   New York
Athens   Auckland   Bangkok   Bogotá   Buenos Aires   Calcutta
Cape Town   Chennai   Dar es Salaam   Delhi   Florence   Hong Kong   Istanbul
Karachi   Kuala Lumpur   Madrid   Melbourne   Mexico City   Mumbai
Nairobi   Paris   São Paulo   Singapore   Taipei   Tokyo   Toronto   Warsaw

and associated companies in
Berlin   Ibadan

Copyright © 1999 by Oxford University Press, Inc.

Published by Oxford University Press, Inc.
198 Madison Avenue, New York, New York 10016

Oxford is a registered trademark of Oxford University Press

Library of Congress Cataloging-in-Publication Data
Nurturing the premature infant :
developmental interventions in the neonatal intensive care nursery /
edited by Edward Goldson.
p. cm.   Includes index.
ISBN 0-19-508570-1
1. Neonatal intensive care.   2. Infants (Premature)—Hospital care.
3. Sensory stimulation in newborn infants.
I. Goldson, Edward.
[DNLM: 1. Infant, Premature—physiology.   2. Infant, Premature, Diseases—therapy.
3. Infant, Low Birth Weight—physiology.   4. Intensive Care Units, Neonatal.
WS 410 N974 1999]   RJ253.5.N875 1999   618.92'011—dc21
DNLM/DLC   for Library of Congress   98-7850

9 8 7 6 5 4 3 2 1

Printed in the United States of America
on acid-free paper.

Foreword

LULA O. LUBCHENCO

Nurturing the Premature Infant is a book about the environment in the neonatal intensive care unit (NICU) and addresses the need for developmental interventions. All of the authors remind us that the premature infant is an individual who needs specialized care based on his or her present level of neurologic development—the ideal aim of all pediatric care. So why are some of these interventions considered controversial? The primary reason is the intensity of care often necessary to save lives. Do NICU interventions interfere with the medical care being given? Is it possible to integrate them into the essential NICU activities? There is also a question of the importance of developmental interventions. The advances in NICU technology have been shown to reduce mortality; will these interventions improve upon the results already achieved? Another reason for the delay in accepting and instituting changes in nursery practices is that the developmental needs of the premature infant, until recently, had not been defined and there were no adequate data about the development of ever smaller preterm infants. Research is still limited, but there is more knowledge upon which to build developmental intervention. Furthermore, there were few convincing data to suggest that changing the nursery environment could have a beneficial effect on long-or short-term outcome.

The chapters in this book speak to these questions. Each author gives an hypothesis for the intervention, and each has designed clinical studies to test the hypothesis. Data from these studies show a beneficial effect on patient outcome. Some of the authors, such as Als, take a holistic approach to infant care, incorporating many interventions, whereas others limit the study to a single procedure. Exactly how these data will be used is not clear, but NICU caregivers have many choices or combinations of measures that may meet their own interests or situations.

For those of us who have watched preterm infants asleep and awake, during feedings and other procedures and have wondered what their various behaviors meant, we now have, in this volume, a guide for observations as well as interpretation of various behaviors. Subtle or overt signs of distress are described. Developmental stages are beginning to be defined and the need for specific stimuli, or avoidance of stimuli, is presented. We can begin to understand the infants' language, so to speak, and can recognize the conditions that lead to distress and those measures that can contribute to the patients' comfort and organization.

Although the importance of maternal bonding was first shown to be vital to the well-being of the infant by the Stanford group, it was Klaus and Kennell who publicized this aspect of newborn care and the need to extend early contact of parents with their fragile preterm infants in the NICU. Interventions given by parents, such as kangaroo care, fulfill a need for both infant and parent.

We should also keep in mind Ramey's observation, in this book, that intervention initiated in the nursery must be continued after discharge. The long-term outcome of the child depends on the caregivers' ability to recognize and respond to the infant. The interventions that include the parents, or caregivers, are of utmost importance.

As the neurologic development of the infant begins to dictate the way in which nursing and medical care is administered, the interventions described in these pages may become routine. When we understand and recognize the stresses to the infant caused by necessary medical and nursing procedures, we will try to lessen the pain by comfort measures before and after the procedure, just as we comfort a child receiving an immunization.

Developmental care, translated as appropriate care for a particular age, is good for the patient, facilitates the healing process, shortens hospital stay, and promotes future development. Perhaps it is the breakthrough neonatal medicine seeks. This volume contains the information necessary to accomplish this breakthrough in the care of the premature infant.

Preface

In contrast to the gestation of the infant discussed in this edited volume, the gestation of this book has been quite prolonged. This volume grew out of discussions with colleagues in medicine and developmental psychology over several years and in reviewing the literature on neonatal interventions. Through these explorations I came to realize that there were many scattered articles and chapters but no single resource that clinicians and researchers could turn to for information. Colleagues confirmed my perception and encouraged me to bring together, in one volume, the more interesting and, perhaps, controversial interventions for which there were available research data and clinical applications. As a result, I have chosen several interventions that are not routinely used in neonatal intensive care units (NICUs) but that have elicited considerable interest among developmental psychologists, developmental pediatricians, and neonatal nurses. Thus, this book is directed toward a wide audience of people involved in the care of the sick infant. By bringing together, under one cover, a discussion of these interventions, we hope that clinicians will be stimulated to consider using these approaches in their units. At the same time, one must recognize that more information is needed about these interventions and their effect on different populations of premature infants. Thus, the authors and I hope that basic scientists will be stimulated to investigate more thoroughly the efficacy of these interventions and to identify the mechanisms by which positive outcomes are achieved.

The books opens with a discussion of the NICU environment. A rather bleak picture is painted of this environment, yet it does reflect what has been described in the literature. Clearly some NICUs have begun to address some of these adverse environmental conditions. Nevertheless, in many nurseries conditions continue to be less than optimal for the staff and infants alike. Chapter 1 is included to highlight the conditions under which the interventions described in this volume are utilized.

The succeeding chapter discusses the developmental interventions that can be employed in the NICU and integrated into the ongoing medical care required by sick infants. Als describes the individualized care plan, which serves as an umbrella for many other interventions. The thrust here is for the caretaker to acknowledge the individual infant's unique needs and to provide developmentally appropriate interventions that are modified according to the infant's physiological and behavioral responses and cues.

Chapter 3, by Ramey and Shearer, presents a theoretical framework for conceptualizing risk and early intervention during and after the NICU hospitalization. They consider risk as a probabilistic concept that includes reproductive and caretaking casualty. They posit that risk can be changed by the family resources as well as by the nature of the care provided and the environment in which it occurs. Ramey and Shearer emphasize the poor fit between the NICU and the infant's needs, thus advocating for the use of individualized care for the infant. Furthermore, they emphasize the need to include parents in the care of the child and to consider the long-term implications of such interventions.

In the remaining chapters, Anderson provides the history and rationale for the use of "kangaroo care," an intervention that can be used in varied situations and settings. She also presents data suggesting this intervention is safe and also facilitates parent-infant interaction.

Korner, Thoman, and Field consider three very specific interventions that seek to enhance the infant's neurobehavioral organization. Korner has been, and continues to be, an advocate for the use of vestibular stimulation through the use of the oscillating water bed. She presents data supporting the efficacy of this intervention for enhancing physiologic organization in the more stable infant. Thoman addresses the infant's capacity for entrainment using a "breathing bear." She argues that with this intervention, in the stable premature infant, neurobehavioral organization and interactional capacities are enhanced. Furthermore, she argues, the infant has more control over his or her environment. Field has recently reopened the field of infant massage. She describes the impact of massage and its efficacy in enhancing neurobehavioral organization. Moreover, she argues that there are considerable advantages to the caretakers who perform this intervention.

The closing chapter presents an overview of the models and interventions described in the book. It discusses some of the clinical implications of these interventions and raises a number of research questions.

This book is directed toward a wide readership that includes physicians, nurses, therapists, and behavioral scientists of many disciplines. It is conceived as a first attempt to bring to this audience developmental interventions that can facilitate and enhance the establishment of the neurobehavioral organization in the sick newborn. The field of developmentally based interventions in the NICU is emerging. The authors and I hope that the information gathered here will stimulate further research into developmental interventions, their mechanisms of action and the nature of their efficacy and will expand their clinical applications.

Denver, Colorado   E. G.
July 1998

Contents

Contributors

HEIDELISE ALS, PH.D.
Department of Psychiatry
Harvard Medical School
    and Children's Hospital
Boston, Massachusetts

GENE CRANSTON ANDERSON, PH.D., R.N.
Frances Payne Bolton School of Nursing
Case Western Reserve University
Cleveland, Ohio

TIFFANY FIELD, PH.D.
Touch Research Institute
Nova Southeastern University
Ft. Lauderdale, Florida

EDWARD GOLDSON, M.D. (EDITOR)
Children's Hospital
    and the University of Colorado
Health Sciences Center
Department of Pediatrics
Denver, Colorado

ANNELIESE F. KORNER, PH.D.
Division of Child Psychiatry
    and Child Development

Stanford University School of Medicine
Stanford, California

LUBA O. LUBCHECO, M.D.
The University of Colorado
Health Sciences Center
Denver, Colorado

CRAIG T. RAMEY, PH.D.
Civitan International Research Center
University of Alabama at Birmingham
Birmingham, Alabama

DARLENE L. SHEARER, PH.D.
Civitan International Research Center
University of Alabama at Birmingham
Birmingham, Alabama

ANNE MILLER SOSTEK, PH.D.
Chief. Behavioral and Social Science IRG
Center for Scientific Review
National Institutes of Health
Bethesda, Maryland

EVELYN B. THOMAN, PH.D
Behavioral Sciences Graduate Program
University of Connecticut
Storrs, Connecticut

Nurturing the Premature Infant

1

THE ENVIRONMENT OF THE NEONATAL INTENSIVE CARE UNIT

EDWARD GOLDSON

In the United States during 1993, about 3,979,000 infants were born. Of this number 7.2%—that is, about 288,482 babies—had birthweights less than 2,500 g (Guyer et al., 1995). The proportion of very low birthweight (VLBW) babies, those weighing less than 1,500 g, was 1.3% in 1993. If one considers the more precise vital statistics from 1990, during which the number of births was 4,158,212, 7%, or 289,419, had a birthweight less than 2,500 g (Monthly Vital Statistics Report, 1993). Of this number, 108,003, or 2.6% of the total number of infants born, had birthweights less than 2,000 g and most likely required some care in a neonatal intensive care unit (NICU). These numbers, however, do not include infants born at term with a variety of birth defects or term infants who sustained severe birth asphyxia and also required intensive care. Thus, the numbers probably underestimate the actual number of infants cared for in NICUs. These infants, who are the sickest, often the smallest, and the most fragile of newborns born in the United States, have a wide variety of prenatal and neonatal difficulties ranging from extreme prematurity and respiratory distress, which can result in intracranial hemorrhage and bronchopulmonary dysplasia, to birth asphyxia leading to hypoxic-ischemic encephalopathy. Many of them also have a variety of life-threatening birth defects. Each of these infants is unique as a result of their individual genetic constitutions, their prenatal and perinatal experiences, and their family's individuality. However, all of these infants have one thing in common—namely, their early life in a NICU. The purpose of this chapter is to describe the environment in which these extremely sick and fragile infants are treated and where their families must make their initial contact with the infant.

There are approximately 750 NICUs in the United States, and in 1991 approximately 3,000 physicians were practicing neonatology (Silverman, 1993). By and large, these units are staffed by highly trained neonatologists and neonatal nurses and are supported by occupational therapists, physical therapists, respiratory therapists, psychologists, social workers, pastoral care workers and a wide variety of medical and surgical specialists. All of these professionals are committed to the survival of the infant and to optimizing each child's medical and developmental outcome. Yet they function and perform their work in environments that may not be conducive to their own well-being (Marshall & Kasman, 1980; White-Traut et al., 1994) or to the well-being of the infants they are committed to caring for.

The intrauterine environment is "designed" to support and nurture the human embryo and fetus. The immature organism floats in the amniotic fluid, a salt solution that is essentially a gravity-free environment, and bumps gently against the uterine walls. Under most circumstances a fetus has all his nutritional and physiologic needs met without expending any excess energy. He is well oxygenated and receives all of his nutrition through the placenta, while his wastes are eliminated by the mother. Moreover, he is sustained in warm, muted, and protected surroundings. A fetus is exposed to a day/night cycle and to soft light that passes through the mother's abdomen. He can hear his mother's heartbeat, her voice, the sounds of her intestinal movements, and the sound of blood flowing through the uterine vessels. Sounds from the extrauterine world can be heard in the womb, yet are muted by the abdominal wall, the uterus, the amniotic fluid, and by the mother's own physiologic sounds. A fetus is vestibularly and proprioceptively stimulated by his mother's movements as he floats in the amniotic fluid.

In contrast, newborn infants, particularly the prematurely born infants who are the focus of this discussion, must live in a neonatal intensive care nursery, where they may receive nutrition through a nasogastric tube or a vein that has been punctured by a needle. They may be encouraged to nipple feeds before they are physiologically ready to perform that task and before their gastrointestinal tracts are mature enough to digest and absorb the nutrients. Oxygen needs may be met through a nasal or oral tube connected to a ventilator that, under the most intrusive conditions, is set to breathe for the infant at a precise rate or, at best, is triggered by the baby's own respiratory efforts. Moreover, these infants may need to be restrained for fear they will disconnect themselves from the ventilator or cause an intravenous line to malfunction. To stay warm, an infant may be placed in an incubator whose temperature and humidity are controlled by an audible motor, or on an open, warmed bed where he is easily accessible to medical and nursing personnel. In this setting the infant is exposed to the glare of fluorescent lights or bright sunlight before his vision can adequately accommodate to these strong stimuli. He is also exposed to sounds of varying intensities, loud human voices, and unmuted random noise, including alarms. Each baby is handled and examined by human hands, and poked by needles. Only rarely is the infant in NICU cuddled. Instead, most interactions with caretakers are confined to often aversive procedures that do not consider the child's physiologic state or readiness to interact with his environment. Finally, he exists in an environment with few contingent responses to his physiologic and behavioral cues. That is to say, the infant is exposed to stimuli or procedures to which he may not be ready or able to adapt.

However, the human fetus and premature infant, despite an often tenuous grasp on life, has a repertoire of behavioral and physiologic capabilities. At 24 weeks a fetus can bring his hands to his mouth and make sucking and swallowing movements. By 28 weeks the coordination of these movements is adequate for oral feeding (Bu'Lock, Woodridge, & Baum, 1990; Goldson, 1987; Volpe, 1995). Gardner & Lubchenco (1998) note that, "[a]lthough isolated components of feeding behavior are all present before 24 weeks gestational age, they are not effectively coordinated for oral feedings before 32–34 weeks gestational age. Coordination of respiration with sucking and swallowing during bottle feeding is consistently achieved by infants >37 weeks post conceptional age" (Bu'Lock et al., 1990). After more than 5 weeks of intrauterine life, a fetus can hear sounds and is able to respond to those stimuli (Sound Study Group, in press). At 24–30 weeks of gestational age, a fetus develops synchronous and conjugate eye movements (Birnholz, 1981). Also at this age a fetus will tighten his lids in response to a bright light. By 30–34 weeks a fetus's eyes open and fixate briefly and the lids close immediately when presented with a bright light (Glass, 1993). By 15 weeks gestation a fetus is sensitive to tactile stimulation and capable of responding to being touched and stroked (Glass, 1994). However, because of neurodevelopmental immaturity the fetus is unable, until 32–34 weeks, to coordinate autonomic responses (heart rate and respirations) when stimulated by such stimuli (Prechtl et al., 1979; Rose, 1983; Volpe, 1995). That is the synchrony between breathing, sucking, and swallowing is poorly developed in the premature infant such that oral feedings, for example, can be difficult and indeed dangerous because of the risk of aspiration. In short, a fetus is well adapted to living in the intrauterine environment yet is unprepared to meet the demands of the extrauterine world into which he is thrust when born prematurely.

Over the years there has been debate about whether infants are understimulated or overstimulated in the NICU (Cornell & Gottfried, 1976). However, there now appears to be a consensus that the two extremes coexist (Lucey, 1977). The infant is bombarded with aversive stimuli: loud noise, bright lights, vigorous handling (overstimulation). Lawson, Daum, & Turkewitz (1977) performed a time-sample every 15 minutes in both the intensive care and grower rooms of an NICU by recording nonspeech sounds, handling, illumination levels, and sound pressure levels. They found that the density of environmental events to which the premature infant was exposed exceeded the stimuli an infant would experience even in a reasonable home environment. Similar NICU conditions were also described by Wolke (1987) and Avery & Glass (1989). However, these stimuli are noncontingent—that is unrelated to cues from the infant,—random, aversive, and essentially meaningless in terms of the infant's developmental level.

LIGHT

As noted above, a fetus is exposed to some light—approximately 2% of incident light passes into the uterine cavity (Glass, 1994). This light also has a diurnal variation associated with a mother's rhythms. The level of illumination recommended for an office in which adults are working is 40–50 foot-candles (ftc) (Glass et al., 1985). In contrast, light levels to which a premature infant is exposed in the NICU exceed those levels five-to tenfold (i.e., 50–90 ftc with levels often over 220 ftc). If the infant happens to be in direct sunlight, peak measurements may be over 1,000 ftc. Other sources of light to which an infant may be exposed include bilirubin lights, heating lamps, and the indirect ophthalmoscope. Light intensity from these sources ranges from 250 to 2000 ftc (Glass, 1988; Lotas, 1992).

What is of considerable concern is the continuous and intense nature of the light exposure and the immaturity of the infant's eye (Robinson & Fiedler, 1992). Preterm infants are at increased risk for retinopathy of prematurity (ROP), a proliferative vascular disease of multifactorial origin that is associated with immaturity of the retina. There is general agreement that this disorder is associated with the effect of elevated levels of oxygen on immature retinal vessels. Taking into consideration the effect of light on the immature retina, Glass and coworkers (1985) have suggested that prolonged exposure to elevated levels of light is associated with an even greater incidence of ROP in very immature infants. However, Fiedler et al. (1992), while identifying that the most immature infants are exposed to the greatest level of illumination, were unable to draw a causal relationship between light and ROP. Nevertheless, they suggest that light in conjunction with other factors could be contributing to the development of ROP. Further studies involving intensity and duration of light exposure; retinal blood flow; the pattern and frequency of eyelid opening; the nature of the cornea, aqueous, and lens; gestational age; and birthweight are needed to clarify the extent to which prolonged, intense light exposure in the premature infant increases the risk for the development of ROP (Robinson & Fielder, 1992b).

The effect of light on the neurological development of the visual system and the capacity of an infant to process visual stimuli also need to be considered. A compromise in the development of visual perception can have a negative effect on later learning and tasks requiring an intact competent visual system. In addition, some data suggest that exposure to continuous high-intensity light, as opposed to exposure to dark/light cycles, is stressful for the small infant, affecting feeding, sleeping, respiratory and pulse rates, oxygenation status, and activity cycles (Lotas, 1992). The long-term sequelae of these effects remain to be determined.

Another issue is the effect of continuous, intense light exposure on rapid eye movement (REM) sleep and on the organization of sleep. Apnea can have deleterious effects on an immature infant's central nervous system (CNS), thus potentially compromising later development (Graven et al., 1992a, 1992b). Also, in the visually impaired, delays are frequently seen in the development of motor milestones, exploratory behavior, and language (Glass, 1993).

A final issue to consider is the effect of bright light on an infant's capacity for social interaction. It is known that preterm infants are able to fix and follow as early as 28 weeks, although they may become apneic as a result. Moreover, when an infant is continually exposed to bright light, there is a tendency toward less eye opening, visual fixing, and tracking and more avoidant behavior, with a resulting decrease in visual contact with caretakers and the environment in general (Hack, Mostow, & Miranda, 1976). Thus, it is suggested that caretakers may engage in less meaningful and contingent interaction with an infant as they experience less visual feedback and more avoidance (Glass, 1993).

The long-term effects of these seemingly aversive experiences remain to be seen. There seem, however, to be negative short-term consequences that might be avoided. Thus, to minimize the potential adverse effects of prolonged, unvarying light exposure, approaches should be developed to protect the infant from these stimuli (Lotas, 1992.)

NOISE

Loud, random, noncontingent, unpatterned noise is another stimulus to which an immature infant is exposed in the NICU. Lawson, Daum, & Turkewitz (1977) and Thomas (1989) documented that sound levels in both the intensive care and grower sections of the NICU were comparable to those produced by traffic on a street corner or the noise inside a bus. Other authors (Gottfried, Hodgman, & Brown, 1984; Graven et al., 1992a, 1992b) have described the presence of intermittent noise such as loud voices, banging incubator doors, pagers, intercoms, monitors, and alarms that can generate levels of 120 dB of noise intensity, which is comparable to the sound of heavy machinery and is more than twice as loud as what would be acceptable for an incubator or for adult exposure in the workplace. Anagnostakis et al. (1980) recorded very high noise levels both within and outside the incubator when the infant was ventilated or was receiving supplemental oxygen. Indeed, the authors found these noise levels had a high probability of affecting sleep even in adults. In relation to other environmental sounds comparable to those in the NICU, 50 dB is roughly the intensity of sound generated by light traffic and 90 dB is equivalent to that generated by light machinery. Industrial standards limit noise exposure to 90 dB for 8 continuous hours a day and 93 dB for 4 continuous hours a day (Graven et al., 1992a, 1992b) (Table 1.1).

Taking the aforementioned data into consideration, consider the effect the noise levels in the nursery might have on an immature auditory system and brain. Moreover, the noise levels in the NICU are the same during the day and night, and, as with light exposure, the infant has no control over or escape from noise exposure (Berens & Weigle, 1995; Nzama, Nolte, & Dorfling, 1995). Thus, NICU noise is essentially a noncontingent, unpatterned, developmentally inappropriate stimulus.

Are there deleterious effects to noise exposure? The most striking short-term effect of NICU noise was described by Long, Lucey, & Philip (1980), who reported the association between loud, sudden noise and agitation and crying in infants, which was related to hypoxemia and an increase in intracranial pressure. Although the relationship between hypoxemia and apnea was not evaluated in this study, there is a known association between these two events, resulting in neonatal morbidity that can have long-term adverse effects on an infant. Potential long-term sequelae of constant noise exposure include an increased risk of sensory hearing loss and abnormal auditory development. Thus,

Table 1.1. Noise Levels in the NICU

Level (dB)	Comments
50–60	Normal speaking voice
50–73.5*†	Incubator (motor noise)
45–85‡	Noise in NICU (talking, equipment alarms, telephones, radio)
48–69	Humidifiers and nebulizers
65–80†	Life support equipment (ventilator, IV pumps)
85	Noise level at which hearing damage is possible for adult; (?) neonatal effects
90§	Adult exposure for 8 hours requires protective device and hearing conservation program
92.8†	Opening incubator porthole
96–117†	Placing bottle of formula on top of incubator
110–116†	Closing one or both cabinet doors
114–124†	Closing one or both portholes
130–140†	Banging incubator to stimulate apneic premature infant
160–165	Recommendations for peak, single noise level not to exceed to prevent (adult) hearing loss; (?) neonatal effects

*American Academy of Pediatrics recommends incubator noise not to exceed 58 dB (Modern incubators generate 51–52 dB).

†Measures from inside the incubator.

‡Noise levels do not vary from morning to night.

§Occupational Safety and Health Administration (OHSA) standard. (No safety standards for neonates have been established.)

Modified from Mitchell SA: *Semin Hear* 5(1):17, 1984.

Reprinted with permission from Merenstein & Gardner (1998).

an issue to raise is the effect of noise on the development of auditory perception and on subsequent learning.

Many prenatal factors and perinatal medical complications contribute to deficits in developmental outcome for infants born prematurely (Goldson, 1996). Nevertheless, the effect of the NICU environment must also be considered in optimizing the development of a prematurely born infant. To see how altering the light and noise environment of the NICU might affect the infant, Mann et al. (1986) reported some provocative results. By decreasing the intensity of light and noise in the nursery and by establishing a night/day cycle, they found that the infants slept more, spent less time feeding, and gained more weight after discharge than matched controls for whom this environmental manipulation had not been instituted.

SOCIAL

In addition to the physical environment of the NICU, it is essential to consider an infant's interactional and caretaking experiences, which may be even more important than the effects of the physical environment. Gottfried, Wallace-Lande, & Sherman-Brown, (1981) evaluated the physical and social environment of infants in a NICU and in a convalescent care nursery. They replicated the work of Lawson, Daum, & Turkewitz (1977) and also demonstrated that the infant received relatively infrequent coordinated sensory experiences with virtually no diurnal rhythmicity. Of particular significance was the fact that handling the infant was primarily related to medical or nursing care and was linked to work schedules and procedures rather than in response to infant behavior. It is reported that in a 2-week period an infant might be cared for and handled by more than 10 different nurses in addition to physicians, respiratory therapists, laboratory and radiology technicians, and occupational and physical therapists (Glass, 1994). The possible negative effects of multiple caretakers include inconsistency of care as well as a lack of understanding of the individual infant's characteristics, behavioral cues, and upsets in feeding and sleeping patterns. This can lead to the infant becoming more stressed and disorganized with resulting physiologic instability and poor weight gain (Cartlett & Holditch-Davis, 1990)

As a means of further evaluating the infant's NICU social experiences, that is to say, interactions with the infant that were independent of medical intervention, Gottfried (1985) studied the environments of a NICU and a neonatal convalescent care unit (NCCU). First, he did a time-sampling analysis of the physical and social environment and found that the infants were exposed to a variety of stimuli and so received considerable sensory stimulation. He also found that these infants had negligible social experiences, such as caretakers rocking and talking gently to the infants and responding to their behavioral cues. In a second study, he looked more closely at the contacts between caregivers and the infants in both the NICU and the NCCU. He found that, in the NICU, there was a greater frequency of medical-nursing care while in the NCCU there was a relatively higher frequency of social events. However, caregivers in both units tended not to respond to infants' cries. Furthermore, there was no difference in the frequency of contacts among the work shifts. Finally, although sensory-integrated experiences of a social nature occurred more often in the NCCU than the NICU, they were not plentiful in either unit. Actual integrated sensory experiences were usually in the context of rocking and social touching, which were minimal. These data demonstrated that the majority of the infants' experiences grew out of medical-care needs, rather than in response to the infants' behavioral cues. As a result, the infants' interactions with the environment were noncontingent and unpredictable.

Linn et al. (1985a) also provided an ecological description of the NICU. The authors maintained that the NICU environment could significantly influence an infant's developmental outcome. They acknowledged that the NICU is designed to provide medical support for the sick infant and that medical interventions are provided for the treatment of well-documented biological disorders that put the infant's life and well-being at risk. However, they argued, echoing the work of Cornell and Gottfried (1976), that most environmental interventions are based on undocumented assumptions about infants' needs. Linn et al. (1985b) studied two different nurseries in the same institution, one crowded and one more spacious. In their study of the two NICUs they continuously recorded a variety of infant, caregiver, and background variables including infant state, infant visual and social behavior, proximity of caregiver to infant, type of background sounds, and a description of toys and mobiles an infant might look at. When an inter-action began, they recorded the type of caregiver attention, the identity of the caregiver, and the nature of the caregiver's tactile, visual, and vocal stimulation of the infant. They found no differences between the NICU settings for any of the variables and concluded that other differences reflected variations in staff behavior rather than in physical setting. With further analyses, they found the amount of time the staff spent in social interactions with an infant was not related to staff-infant ratios but rather to infant characteristics or staff perception of the importance of social contact.

When relationships with preterm infants in the NICU were compared to term infants in their homes, Linn et al. (1985) found that term infants were exposed to less adult speech and the crying of other infants. The term infants were exposed to much less nonspecific activity and sounds, invariant mechanical sounds, and nonspecific activity sounds. They were exposed to more vestibular stimulation and to more gentle touching and vestibular stimulation (gentle rock-ing) than were the premature infants in the nursery. The term infants vocalized more, cried more, and looked at the caregiver more frequently than did the preterm babies in the NICU. The amount of interaction the preterm infants had with caretakers was a function of the infants' initial medical complications and degree of prematurity rather than their current state of health. The level of contingent responsivity of caregivers—that is, the caregivers' response to the infants' cues rather than the caregivers' medical attention—was variable. Infants who did display vocal and visual behaviors received caregivers' contingent re-sponses. However, it must be noted that a significant number of these stable infants did not respond to their caregivers even when appropriately stimulated.

Eckerman et al. (1996) identified differences between VLBW infants and term infants in their affect during face-to-face interactions with their mothers and with unfamiliar female adults when the infants were 4 months corrected age and out of the nursery. The VLBW infants showed significantly less positive affect than did the healthy term infants.

The behavior identified by Linn et al. (1985) and Eckerman et al. (1996) may be one of the outcomes of living in the NICU, or it may be a reflection of an infant's immature central nervous system. Nevertheless, it is apparent from these studies that the NICU is not like a home environment, which does not bombard the infant with physical stimuli and is usually far more responsive to an infant's demands. Although there was some individualized care in the NICU, an infant's day depended, usually, on the nursery schedule and not on his cues. Infants in the NICU likely are not understimulated but instead may be bombarded by "meaningless" stimuli in a rather nonsocial environment that provides little con-tingent physical and social stimulation (Bennett, 1987; Gottfried & Hodgman, 1985). Thus, they are "deprived" of meaningful sensory and social experiences. In earlier studies Eckerman et al. (1994, 1995) identified differences between high-and low-risk infants with birthweights <1,500 g in their attention and abil-ity to modulate their responses to social interactions. The sicker babies had considerably more difficult times than did the healthier infants. The results revealed by the Eckerman et al. study (1996) suggest that this infant behavior may be a prolonged effect of the NICU experience or the result of prematurity itself.

PROCEDURES

Another aspect of the handling and interactions between the infant and the caretakers that needs to be considered is the physical effect of medical procedures on the infant. Using continuous transcutaneous monitoring, Long, Philip, & Lucey (1980) studied low birthweight infants during their stay in the NICU. Through this study they sought to (1) quantitate the amount of hypoxemia or hyperoxemia the infants experienced; (2) define the relationship, if any, between intensive care procedures and abnormalities of oxygenation; and (3) determine whether hypoxemia or hyperoxemia could be eliminated by using transcutaneous oxygen monitoring to modify practices in the NICU. Infants in the NICU were subjected to repetitive diagnostic, nursing, and therapeutic procedures performed with little attention to the infant's physiologic and behavioral state and resulted in undetected episodes of hypoxemia or hyperoxemia. Indeed, 75% of the episodes of hypoxemia experienced by the infants were associated with handling by NICU personnel, and only 5% of these episodes were evidenced by apnea and bradycardia. By using the transcutaneous monitor during nursery procedures, these investigators were able to demonstrate that, as the quality of handling the infant improved, the number of hypoxic episodes dramatically decreased. Murdoch & Darlow (1984) reported similar findings of hypoxemia in association with suctioning and handling in the NICU. Moreover, they found that infants undergoing intensive care were handled an average of 18% in a 24-hour period and received an average of 234 handling procedures during that time period. Many procedures were associated with undesirable consequences such as hypoxemia. Parental handling occurred 35% of the time but was usually benign and did not result in this physiologic stress. Handling procedures definitely interfered with the infants' rest and represented intrusions over which the infants had no control.

Another study that evaluated the effect of a nursing procedure, by Perlman and Volpe (1983), sought to determine the relationship between suctioning and changes in the cerebral circulation. The authors found a prominent increase in cerebral blood flow velocity associated with suctioning, which was accompanied by increased blood pressure and increased intracranial pressure. These changes in cerebral blood circulation place the very sick and fragile infant at increased risk for intracranial hemorrhage and its developmental consequences. These findings have been replicated by the work of Shah et al. (1992), who found that with endotracheal suctioning arterial hemoglobin saturation and brain intravascular hemoglobin saturation decreased and cerebral blood volume increased. These findings confirmed that endotracheal suctioning was associated with a transient hypoxemia, which is reflected in cerebral vasodilation and deoxygenation. In the VLBW and very immature infant, these alterations in oxygenation place the infant at high risk for cerebral disturbances. These effects, according to these authors, are preventable by preoxygenation prior to suctioning.

Hypoxemia, apnea, and bradycardia are the most striking responses that the preterm infant may have to stress. When these events occur, the infant has been significantly disturbed. Based on clinical observations of VLBW infants with no major perinatal complications, Gorski (1983), Gorski et al. (1983) and High & Gorski (1985) have suggested and demonstrated, using a direct computer recording of the infant, a number of subtle behavioral cues that even the smallest infant provides when stressed. During nursing interventions or social interactions for which the infant is unprepared or is incapable of processing, these infants showed "subtle behavioral distress" characterized by arching of the trunk, gaze aversion, grimacing, and frowning. They further identified "subtle physiologic distress," such as sustained crying, pale or red skin color, hiccups, regurgitation of feeds, and unceasing limb movements. These events often preceded signs of "gross behavioral and physiologic distress," such as mottled or cyanotic skin color, apnea, bradycardia, nasal flaring, or intercostal or subcostal retractions. Through the use of this technology, they support the idea that the infant can be significantly stressed by events perceived by health-care providers as necessary and helpful and show that one needs to closely monitor subtle signs of stress to avoid precipitous physiologic decompensation in the fragile infant.

The time that the premature infant spends in the NICU is a particularly sensitive period when the infant is physiologically fragile and has little control over his physical and emotional environment or over the individuals caring for him. Under normal circumstances, he would still be in the womb protected from the external environment with which he is unprepared to interact. Developmentally, this is also a time when there is considerable neurologic growth, with many of the substrata for later neurodevelopmental processes being laid down. Clearly, the environment of the NICU is very different from the intrauterine environment. I do not suggest, however, that one should argue for or against replicating the intrauterine environment or for stimulating the infant to be able to cope with the extrauterine environment. Instead, I emphasize the fact that there is a debate and that it is essential to recognize not only the strengths but also the limitations of the prematurely born infant and the potential—even probable—deleterious effects of the NICU environment.

Of course, parents deserve attention. With the birth of a premature infant the mother and father are catapulted away from the normal processes of full-term gestation when they would establish a relationship with the unborn infant. Normally, there is time to prepare a place for the baby, to discuss a name, and to begin to separate from the life that existed prior to the infant's arrival. This relationship comes to fruition with the birth or the anticipated birth of a normal infant. Expectant couples are supported by family and friends and "inducted" into the ranks of parents. In contrast, with premature birth, particularly of a sick child, this preparation and happy anticipation is abruptly curtailed. Instead, parents face anxiety, grief, fear, and the need to adapt to an unfamiliar environment. They are "forced" to hand over their infant to strangers, who the parents hope will preserve their infant's life and return to them a healthy baby. This ordeal is extraordinarily stressful for parents and is fraught with risks for the parent-child relationship (Goldson, 1992).

RECOMMENDATIONS

I have attempted here to demonstrate ways in which the NICU can be an aversive setting for a fragile premature infant. Workers involved in the care of such infants need to find ways to change the physical environment and their own behaviors in this setting. Lotas (1992), Graven et al. (1992a, 1992b), and Glass (1994) have made some specific recommendations to this end: Lighting should be reduced in the NICU, and a day/night cycle should be established. One way to accomplish this is to use individual bedside lighting and to dim the lights in the nursery. Another approach to dealing with light, and sound as well, is be to cover the isolette. Noise intensity should be decreased not only in the NICU itself but also in the incubator and other equipment in contact with an infant. Caregivers should interact verbally with each infant on a contingent basis with a patterned interaction and consider the infant's cues, responses, and needs. Since many of the handling procedures and physical interactions are exceedingly stressful, caregivers should be able to read an infant's cues indicating stress and distress and respond to them. Thus, caregivers must be alert and responsive to the needs of the infant, and medical and nursing procedures should be timed to be minimally stressful (Merenstein, 1994). Furthermore, it is important that caregivers recognize that their physical caretaking and social interactions with the infant can have long-term effects, both positive and negative.

A final suggestion that emerges from this review is that NICUs be reorganized to be more compatible with the physiologic and developmental needs of the immature infant. Currently NICUs are organized around a systems model rather than on the care of the individual (Gilkerson, Gorksi, & Panitz, 1990). This approach does not consider the nature and the significance of an individual's relationship to the environment. Thus, the nursery is organized to provide acute care, only, which allows the caretakers to "do their job," rather than around the specific developmental, long-term needs of the infant and family. As a rule, hospitals (and nurseries) do not reach out to address broad environmental, developmental, social, and cultural factors and the effect their organization and care may have on those domains. In a letter to the editor, White (1992) asked why NICUs that are noxious to the infant continue to be built? Among the reasons cited for the current approach to design and construction is the safety of the infant. However, among the reasons may be the convenience of the staff as well as cost and space constraints. Beyond safety, changes may well be needed to enhance the infant's well-being. Svenningsen (1993) supports the idea that improved environmental engineering of the NICU is necessary to improve the outcome of the high-risk infant. Tetlow (1992) described an NICU that incorporated a day/night cycle, low noise, and a home-like design. The efficacy and safety of this setting have yet to be evaluated, but preliminary results suggest that the nursing staff agrees that this kind of environment encourages an infant's well-being.

Whether changes in the construction and organizations of NICUs will occur in the immediate future remains to be seen. There certainly is evidence that changes in the NICU environment that minimize noncontingent, uncoordinated sensory stimulation have a positive effect on the infant. Some such alterations have been made in some NICUs. Meanwhile, caregivers attempting developmental interventions for the premature infant continue to work within systems model environments. The authors contributing to this volume will describe the efficacy, or lack of efficacy, of particular interventions under existing conditions. It is interesting to speculate and advantageous to study whether significant alterations in the physical and caretaking environment of the NICU would enhance the effects of developmental interventions designed to nurture the premature infant and enhance the developmental outcome for these fragile infants. For those data the reader will have to wait for researchers to design the appropriate studies in different NICU settings.

Acknowledgments

Appreciation is extended to Sandy Garnder, RN, for critical review and helpful suggestions in the preparation of this manuscript.

REFERENCES

Advance Report of Final Natality Statistics, 1990. (1993). *Monthly Vital Statistics Report, 41*, no. 9, Supplement. February 25.

Anagnostakis, D., Petmezakis, J., Messaritakis, J., & Matsaniotis, N. (1980). Noise pollution in neonatal units: a potential health hazard. *Acta Paediatrica Sandinavica, 69*, 771–773.

Avery, G. B., & Glass, P. (1989). The gentle nursery: developmental intervention in the NICU. *Journal of Perinatology, 9*, 204–206.

Bennett, F. C. (1987). The effectiveness of early intervention for infants at increased biologic risk. In F. C. Bennett & M. J. Gurlanick (Eds.), *The Effectiveness of Early Intervention for At-risk and Handicapped Children* (pp. 79–112). San Diego: Academic Press.

Berens, R. J., & Weigle, C. G. (1995). Noise measurements during high-frequency oscillatory and conventional mechanical ventilation. *Chest, 108*, 1026–1029.

Birnholz, J. C. (1981). The development on human fetal eye movement patterns. *Science, 213*, 679–681.

Bu'Lock, F., Woodridge, M. W., & Baum, J. D. (1990). Development of coordination of sucking, swallowing, and breathing: ultrasound study of term and preterm infants. *Developmental Medicine and Child Neurology, 32*, 669–678.

Cartlett, A. T., & Holditch-Davis, D. (1990). Environmental stimulation of the acutely ill premature infant: physiologic effects and nursing implications. *Neonatal Network, 8*, 19–26.

Cornell, E. H., & Gottfried, A. W. (1976). Intervention with premature infants. *Child Development, 47*, 32–39.

Eckerman, C. O., Oehler, J. M., Medvin, M. D., & Hannan, T. E. (1994). Premature infants as social partners before term age. *Infant Behavior and Development, 17*, 55–70.

Eckerman, C. O., Oehler, J. M., Hannan, T. E., & Molitor, A. (1995). The development prior to term age of very prematurely born newborns' responsiveness in *en face* exchanges. *Infant Behavior and Development, 18*, 283–297.

Eckerman, C. O., Oehler, J. M., Hsu, H-C., Molitor, A., Gill, K., & Leung, E. (1996). Infants positive affect during *en face* exchanges: Effects of premature birth, race, and social partner. *Infant Behavior and Development, 19*, 435.

Fiedler, A. R., Robinson, J., Shaw, D. E., Ng. Y. K., & Moseley, M. J. (1992). Light and retinopathy of prematurity: does retinal location offer a clue? *Pediatrics, 89*, 648–653.

Gardner, S. L., & Lubchenco, L. O. (1998). The neonate and the environment: impact on development. In G. B. Merenstein & S. L. Gardner (Eds.), *Handbook of Neonatal Intensive Care* (4th ed.). St. Louis: Mosby Year Book.

Gilkerson, L., Gorski, P. A., & Panitz, P. (1990). Hospital-based intervention for preterm infants and their families. In S. J. Meisels & J. P. Shonkoff (Eds.), *Handbook of Early Childhood Intervention* (pp. 445–468). Cambridge: Cambridge University Press.

Glass, P. (1988). Role of light toxicity in the developing retinal vasculature. *Birth Defects: Original Article Series, 24*, 103–117.

Glass, P. (1993). Development of visual function in preterm infants: Implications for early intervention. *Infants and Young Children, 6*, 11–20.

Glass, P. (1994). The vulnerable neonate and the neonatal intensive care environment. In G. B. Avery, M. A. Fletcher, & M. G. MacDonald, *Neonatology: Pathophysiology and Management of the Newborn*, (4th ed., pp. 77–91). Philadelphia: J. B. Lippincott.

Glass, P., Avery, G. B., Subramanian, K. N. S., Keys, M. P., Sostek, A. M., & Friendly, D. S. (1985). Effect of bright light in the hospital nursery on the incidence of retinopathy of prematurity. *New England Journal of Medicine, 313*, 401–404.

Goldson, E. (1987). Nonnutritive sucking in the sick infant. *Journal of Perinatology, 7*, 30–34.

Goldson, E. (1992). The neonatal intensive care unit: premature infants and parents. *Infants and Young Children, 4*, 31–42.

Goldson, E. (1996). Follow-up of low birth weight infants: neurodevelopmental and educational sequelae. In M. L. Wolraich (Ed.), *The Practical Assessment and Management of Children With Disorders of Development and Learning* (2nd ed.). Chicago: Mosby Year Book.

Gorski, P. A. (1983). Premature infant behavioral and physiologic responses to caregiving interventions in the intensive care nursery. In J. D. Call, E. Galenson, & R. L. Tyson (Eds.), *Frontiers in Infant Psychiatry* (pp. 256–263). New York: Basic Books.

Gorski, P. A., Hole, W. T., Leonard, C. H., & Martin, J. A. (1983). Direct computer recording of premature infants and nursery care. *Pediatrics, 72*, 198–202.

Gottfried, A. W. (1985). Environment of newborn infants in special care units. In A. W. Gottfried & J. L. Gaiter (Eds.), *Infant Stress Under Intensive Care* (pp. 23–54). Baltimore: University Park Press.

Gottfried, A. W., Hodgman, J. E., & Brown, K. W. (1984). How intensive is newborn intensive care: an environmental analysis. *Pediatrics, 74*, 292–294.

Gottfried, A. W., Wallace-Lande, P., & Sherman-Brown, S. (1981). Physical and social environment of newborn infants in special care units. *Science, 214*, 637–675.

Graven, S. N., Bowen, F. W., Brooten, D., Eaton, A., et al. (1992a). The high-risk infant environment. Part 1. The role of the neonatal intensive care unit in the outcome of high-risk infants. *Journal of Perinatology, 12,* 164–172.

Graven, S. N., Bowen, F. W., Brooten, D., Eaton, A., et al (1992b). The high-risk infant environment. Part 2. The role of caregiving and the social environment. *Journal of Perinatology, 12,* 267–275.

Guyer, B., Strobino, D. M., Ventura, S. J., & Singh, G. K. (1995). Annual summary of vital statistics—1994. *Pediatrics, 96,* 1029–1039.

Hack, M., Mostow, A., & Miranda, S. B. (1976). Development of attention in preterm infants. *Pediatrics, 58,* 669–674.

High, P. C., & Gorski, P. S. (1985). Womb for improvement—A study of preterm development in an intensive care nursery. In A. W. Gottfried & J. L. Gaiter (Eds.), *Infant Stress Under Intensive Care: Environmental Neonatology* (pp. 131–155). Baltimore: University Park Press.

Lawson, K. W., Daum, C., & Turkewitz, G. (1977). Environmental characteristics of a neonatal intensive-care unit. *Child Development, 48,* 1633–1639.

Linn, P. L., Horowitz, F. D., Buddin, B. J., Leaker, J. C., & Fox, H. A. (1985b). An ecological description of a neonatal intensive care unit. In A. W. Gottfried & J. L. Gaiter (Eds.), *Infant Stress Under Intensive Care: Environmental Neonatology* (pp. 83–111). Baltimore: University Park Press.

Linn, P. L., Horowitz, F. D., & Fox, H. (1985a). Stimulation in the NICU: is more necessarily better? *Clinics in Perinatology, 12,* 407–422.

Long, J. G., Lucey, J., & Philip, A. (1980). Noise and hypoxemia in the intensive care nursery. *Pediatrics, 65,* 83–89.

Long, J. G., Philip, A. G. A. S., & Lucey, J. F. (1980). Excessive handling as a cause of hypoxemia. *Pediatrics, 65,* 203–207.

Lotas, M. J. (1992). Effects of light and sound in the neonatal intensive care unit environment on the low-birth-weight infant. *NAACOG'S Clinical Issues in Perinatal and Women's Health Nursing, 3,* 34–44.

Lucey, J. F. (1977). Is intensive care becoming too intensive? *Pediatrics, 59,* 1064–1065.

Mann, N. P., Haddow, R., Stokes, L., Goodley, S., & Rutter, N. (1986). Effect of night and day on preterm infants in a newborn nursery: randomized trial. *British Medical Journal, 293,* 1265–1267.

Marshall, R. W., & Kasman, C. (1980). Burnout in the neonatal intensive care unit. *Pediatrics, 65,* 1161–1165.

Merenstein, S. L. (1994) Editorial. *Journal of the American Medical Association, 272,* 890.

Murdoch, D. R., & Darlow, B. A. (1984). Handling during neonatal intensive care. *Archives of Disease in Children, 59,* 957–961.

Nzama, N. P., Nolte, A. G., Dorfling, C. S (1995). Noise in a neonatal unit: guidelines for the reduction or prevention of noise. *Curationis, 18,* 16–21.

Perlman, J. M., & Volpe, J. J. (1983). Suctioning in the preterm infant: effects on cerebral blood flow velocity, intracranial pressure, and arterial blood flow. *Pediatrics, 72,* 329–334.

Prechtl, H. F. R., Fargel, J. W., Weinmann, H. M., & Bakker, H. H. (1979). Postures, motility and respiration of low-risk pre-term infants. *Developmental Medicine and Child Neurology, 21,* 3–27.

Robinson, J., & Fiedler, A. R. (1992a). Light and the immature visual system. *Eye, 6,* 166–172.

Robinson, J., & Fiedler, A. R. (1992b). Light and the neonatal eye. *Behavior and Brain Research, 49,* 51–55.

Rose, S. A. (1983). Behavioral and psychophysiological sequelae of preterm-birth: the neonatal period. In T. Field & A. Sostek (Eds.), *Infants Born at Risk: Physiological, Perceptual, and Cognitive Processes* (pp. 45–67). New York: Grune & Stratton.

Shah, A. R., Kurth, C. D., Gwiazdowski, S. G., Chance, G., Delivoria-Papadopoulos, M. (1992). Fluctuations in cerebral oxygenation and blood volume during endotracheal suctioning in premature infants. *Journal of Pediatrics, 120*, 769–774.

Silverman, W. A. (1993). Is neonatal medicine in the United States out of step? *Pediatrics, 92*, 612–613.

Sound Study Group. (In press). The effects of sound, noise and vibration in the environment of the high risk infant. University of South Florida, Tampa.

Svenningsen, N. W. (1993). Neonatal care of very low birth weight pre-term infants in the 1990's in Sweden. *Acta Opthalmologia Supplement, 210*, 27–29.

Tetlow, K. (1992). Neonatal environments. *Interiors, 151*, 94.

Thomas, K. A. (1989). How the NICU environment sounds to a premature infant. *American Journal of Maternal and Child Nursing, 14*, 249–251.

Volpe, J. J. (1995). *Neurology of the Newborn* (3rd ed.). Philadelphia: W. B. Saunders.

White, R. (1992). Design of ICUs [letter]. *Pediatrics, 89*, 1267.

White-Traut, R. C., Nelson, M. N., Burns, K., & Cunningham, N. (1994). Environmental influences on the developing premature infant: theoretical issues and applications to practice. *Journal of Obstetrical and Gynecological Neonatal Nursing, 23*, 393–401.

Wolke, D. (1987). Environmental Neonatology. *Archives of Disease in Childhood, 62*, 987–988.

2

READING THE PREMATURE INFANT

HEIDELISE ALS

> *Parents endow even the smallest movements [of their infant] with
> highly personal meaning and react to them affectively.*
>
> Brazelton, Koslowski, & Main,
> *The Origins of Reciprocity* (1974)

Over the past two decades there has been a marked increase in the survival of low birthweight infants both in the United States and abroad. Of the 3.9 million live births annually in the United States, approximately 7.3% are born at less than 2,500 g and more than 4 weeks too early and approximately 1.3% are born at very low birthweight (VLBW), less than 1,500 g (Guyer et al., 1996). For infants with birthweights between 750 g and 1,000 g, born 14–16 weeks too early, survival is now likely (>50%), and for infants with birthweights between 1,000 g and 1,250 g, it is now probable. More than 95% of infants born about 8–12 weeks too early will live if cared for in a newborn intensive care unit (NICUs) associated with a perinatal referral center. In order not only to assure survival but also to foster best development of the increasing number of preterm infants, an understanding of their functioning and progression is critical. An evolutionary developmental perspective may prove helpful.

Such a perspective sees preterm infants as fetuses who develop in extrauterine settings at a time when their brains are growing more rapidly than at any other time in their life span (McLennan, Gilles, & Neff, 1983). As members of the human species, they require three secure environments to support their development: their mother's womb, their parents' bodies, and their family's and community's social group (Hofer, 1987). While they are organized with such bio- and neurodevelopmental needs, preterm infants are removed from these environments at a highly vulnerable phase of brain development. At the same time they need care available only in technologically specialized medical environments: NICUs and special care nurseries (SCNs). Preterm infants have been shown to be at high risk for organ impairments, the most devastating of which include chronic lung disease or bronchopulmonary dysplasia (BPD); (Avery et al., 1987; O'Brodovich & Mellins, 1985), intraventricular hemorrhage (IVH); Volpe, 1989a, 1989b), retinopathy of prematurity (ROP; Gong et al. 1989), and necrotizing enterocolitis (NEC; Kliegman & Walsh, 1987). Even in the more stable low birthweight infants, whose organs may be spared such dramatic insults, the mismatch of the central nervous system's (CNS) expectations of the intrauterine environment and the demands made on the CNS by the NICU may present significant challenges that influence the infant's neuropsychological, psychoemotional, and psychosocial development (Als, 1992; Hunt, Cooper, & Tooley, 1988; McCormick, 1992). Moreover, the disruption of the usual emotional and physical stages of pregnancy that may influence parental preparation for nurturing the child is exacerbated by the emotional trauma experienced by the parents, adding to the challenge for infant and parents (Als, 1986; Als, 1992; Cupoli et al., 1986; Klaus & Kennel, 1982; Klaus, 1982; Minde et al., 1980; Minde et al., 1978; Minde et al., 1983).

Some scientists still hold that the brain of the very preterm infant is so immature that it does not matter what sensory input the brain is exposed to. Outcome is thought to be biologically determined and not subject to early influence (Hack et al., 1994). This assumption, however, has to be questioned, given that even the medically healthy preterm infant with only a transient need for respiratory support, who is at low risk of developing lung disease or IVH, does not appear to be spared later developmental problems, among them specific learning disabilities, consistently lower intelligence quotients, impaired executive function and attention deficit disorders, lower thresholds of fatigue that may adversely influence many activities of daily living, distractibility, impulsivity, concentration difficulties, visual motor impairments, spatial processing disturbances, language comprehension and speech problems, as well as emotional vulnerability and difficulties with self-regulation and self-esteem (Als et al., 1989; Chaudhari et al., 1991; Duffy, Als & McAnulty, 1990; Hunt, Tooley, & Cooper, 1992; Hunt, Tooley, & Harvin, 1982; Largo et al., 1990; Oberklaid et al., 1991; Sostek, 1992; Waber, McCormick, & Workman-Daniels, 1992). Often, even medically low-risk preterm infants appear to show significant school performance deficits and have increased need for special education services (Sostek, 1992). These developmental vulnerabilities become accentuated when there are parental impairments and poor social circumstances (Liaw & Brooks-Gunn, 1993). From these findings, it appears that preterm infants, even those who are medically at low risk, are largely unprepared for the postbirth adjustments they must make, and their development in the extrauterine environment can lead to different and potentially maladaptive developmental trajectories. Knowledge of the neurodevelopmental needs the fetal infant brings to the extrauterine world might provide a basis for the modification of routine and perhaps often inappropriate care. Thus, as a result of little understanding of an infant's vulnerabilities, the very care designed to support an infant may increase the stress and challenge to the already vulnerable, immature nervous system, thereby compromising the immature child.

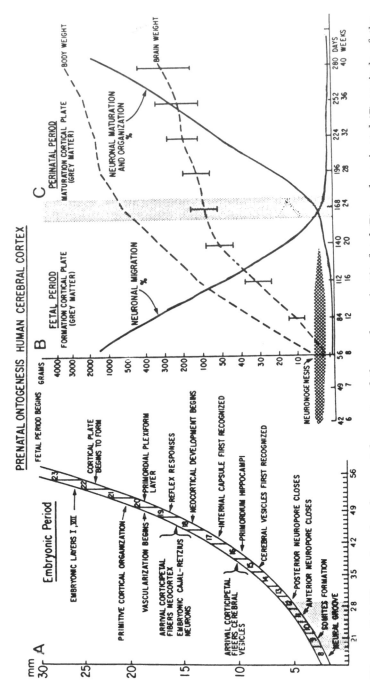

Figure 2.1 The major developmental events of the embryonic (A), fetal (B), and perinatal (C) periods of the prenatal ontogenesis of the human cerebral cortex. The embryonic period is characterized by the appearance of the cerebral vesicles, the arrival of the first corticipetal fibers, and the establishment of the primordial plexiform layer (PPL) prior to the formation of the cortical plate. The fetal period is characterized by the process of neuronal migration and the inside-out formation of the cortical plate. The perinatal period is characterized by the ascending neuronal differentiation and maturation of the cortical plate (gray matter). (Reprinted with permission from Marin-Padilla, 1993)

BRAIN-ENVIRONMENT INTERACTION

The presence of neurodevelopmental impairment in preterm infants spared the insults of intracranial hemorrhage or known hypoxemic/anoxic events suggests that the environment may influence the development of the immature brain in additional ways. Development of the CNS may be influenced by visual, auditory, cutaneous, tactile somasthetic, kinesthetic, olfactory, and gustatory experiences. The complexity and rapidity of fetal brain development, as described by Gilles Leviton, & Dooling (1983), Marin-Padilla (1993), and Rakic (1991), strengthens the hypothesis that the interplay of negative sensory experiences in the womb may lead to malfunction or distortion of brain development and thereby neurobehavioral dysfunction (Duffy et al., 1984). Thus, knowledge of fetal brain development and its dynamic interplay with experience and neurobehavioral functioning will be critical for the better understanding of preterm infant development.

The human cortex begins development around the sixth week of gestation, when the embryo is less than 1.5 cm in length. This occurs with the arrival of primitive corticipetal fibers, followed by the establishment of a superficial primordial premammalian plexiform lamina. Cortical layer I, part of this premammalian plexiform lamina, appears to be necessary for the subsequent inside-out formation of the cortical plate. This represents the basis of the mammalian neocortical gray matter, and appears to play a significant role in the overall structural organization of the mammalian cerebral cortex. It controls the migration of all its future neurons regardless of size, cortical location, or functional role (Marin-Padilla, 1983, 1993). Figure 2.1 schematically presents the early stages of cortical formation. By 6 weeks, the superficial musculature of the embryo is highly developed (Gesell & Armatruda, 1945), as Figure 2.2 shows, and cutaneous innervation and sensitivity become apparent (Humphrey, 1964). As Figure 2.3 shows, this maturation begins with sensitivity about the mouth, including the mucosal skin inside the mouth which extends to the nose and chin, then to the eyelids, palms of the hands, the genitalia, and the soles of the feet. By 12 weeks postmenstrual age, or 10 weeks postovulatory age, the entire face is sensitive. Thus, feedback loops between cutaneous sensitivity, movement, and cortical development are being established early in gestation, dynamically building the vast organization of the highly complex CNS. It is of interest that throughout development, a disproportionately large region of the somatosensory cortex is dedicated to the earliest innervated surface regions, the perioral region, the palms of the hands and the soles of the feet (Figure 2.4; Willis & Grossman, 1981), supporting the exquisitely fine point-to-point discrimination of these regions. It is these regions that appear disproportionately activated yet difficult to inhibit in a prematurely externalized fetus (Als, 1982b). A preterm infant shows foot-bracing, hand and foot grasping, hand-to-mouth efforts, and searching with mouth and tongue while making strong efforts to tuck the trunk into flexion, especially in the first 24–48 hours after delivery (Figures 2.5 and 2.6) (Nilsson, 1973).

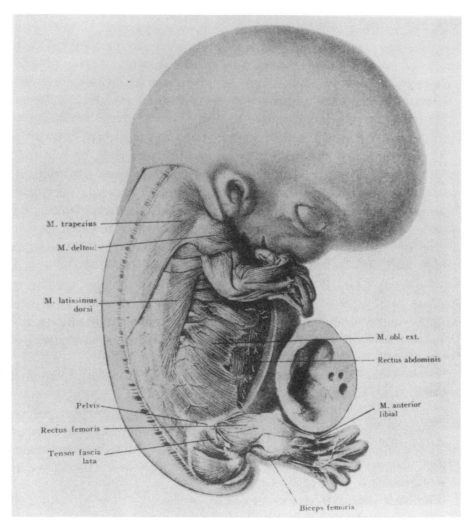

Figure 2.2 Dissection showing the advanced development of the superficial muscles in a 20 mm embryo estimated to be 8 weeks old. (Reprinted with permission from Gesell & Armatruda, 1945)

Denny-Brown's (1966) model of motor system development suggests that gradual differentiation of the dual antagonist integration of avoidance and approach movements underlies all motor system development. The differentiated and complex forward exploratory spontaneous movement repertoire of the fetus has been increasingly documented through ultrasound studies (Birnholz, 1988; de Vries et al., 1985; de Vries, Visser, & Prechtl, 1982, 1988; Hepper & Shahidullah, 1992; Ianniruberto & Tajani, 1981; Tajani & Ianniruberto, 1990; Valman & Pearson, 1980). These studies demonstrate an infant's flexor-extensor

Menstrual Age (Weeks)	Skin Area Sensitive to Stimulation
7.5	About the mouth (perioral)
8–9.5	Alae of the nose and the chin
10–10.5	Eyelids and palms of the hand
10.5	Shoulder
	Genital and anal area
	Genitofemoral sulcus
10.5–11	Soles of the feet
11	Eyebrow and forehead
	Upper arm and forearm
11.5	Entire face
	Upper chest
11–12	Thighs and legs
13	Remaining chest area
14	Tongue, inside of the mouth, all mucous membranes (earlier?)
	Back, side of trunk, and over scapula
15	Abdomen
17	Buttocks

Figure 2.3. Stages of Sensitivity Development. (Reprinted with permission from Humphrey, 1964)

adjustments; complex grasping and release sequences; interaction with the continuously available, pliable, and moving umbilical cord; exploration of face, neck, and head; sucking; holding on with one hand to the other; stepping; clasping one foot against the other, and so forth. This leads one to speculate that these behaviors result in the establishment of increasingly complex feedback loops, characteristic of the human brain.

Each of the millions of neurons in cerebral cortex originates in the germinal lining of the ventricular system. In its prime, the germinal matrix releases as many as 100,000 cortical neurons per day, each of which migrates through the entire thickness of cortex to specific locations (Dooling, Chi, & Gilles, 1983). These migrations occur in waves, beginning, as mentioned, at around 8 postovulatory weeks and gradually tailing off around 24 weeks of pregnancy (Figure 2.1b), when neuronal maturation and organization increases dramatically (Figure 2.1c). Since infants born at 24 weeks gestational age currently have a survival rate outside the womb of about 50%, much of this neuronal maturation and organization occurs for preterm infants in the interaction with an evolutionarily unexpected extrauterine environment. Each of the estimated trillion human neurons, once having migrated to their respective locations, develops dendritic and axonal interconnections with an average of 100 other cells, yielding an estimated quintillion synapses. While the first synaptic contacts are established as early as 7 weeks gestation (Larroche, 1981), new cortical cells are probably generated at

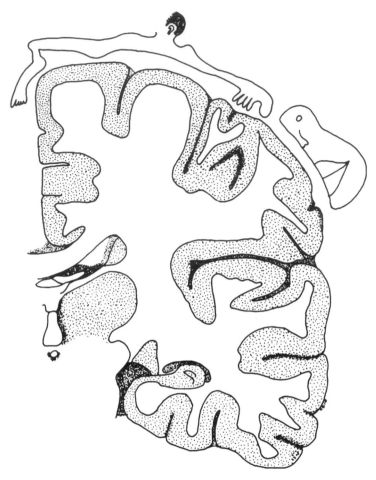

Figure 2.4 The area of the somatosensory cortex that is devoted to the representation of the various parts of the body surface is indicated by a distorted drawing of the human body, known as a sensory homunculus. More cortical tissue is devoted to the face and hand than to other parts of the body; thus, these regions are proportionately larger in the homunculus. (Reprinted with permission from Willis & Grossman, 1981)

a low rate up until and beyond 40 weeks. Synapses continue to be richly established until a child reaches 5 years of age and, more slowly, at least until 18 years of age.

As cells become larger and more elaborately connected, more sulci and gyri develop with different areas organizing for different functions (Cowan & Thoresen, 1985; Springate, 1981). A marked increase in the number of gyri occurs at the end of the second trimester, correlating with a growth spurt of the brain in terms of weight (Gilles, 1983; Marin-Padilla, 1993) and a change in head contour from oval to prominent biparietal prominence (Gilles, 1983). At this

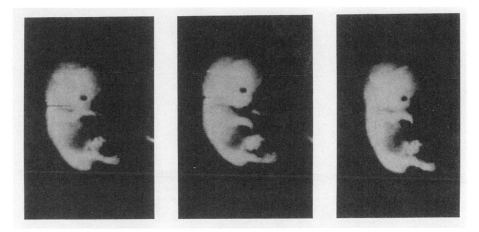

Figure 2.5 The earliest recorded fetal movement. The fetus (crown-rump length, 25 mm) is estimated to be 8.5 weeks old. (Reprinted with permission from Gesell & Armatruda, 1945)

time fetal behavior becomes increasingly complex with increased sucking on fingers or hand; grasping, extension, and flexion rotations; increasingly discernible sleep and wake periods; and reactions to sound.

Another important developmental process that occurs is myelination, which involves the development of a fatty sheath, somewhat like insulation, which is deposited around the axons and allows for more rapid and highly repetitive conduction of impulses. Myelination is thought to accommodate the increased length of the neuronal tracks with growth (Springate, 1981). Myelination seems to occur with peak activity around full-term birth, but continues until 9 years of age and lasts perceptibly into one's forties (Leviton & Gilles, 1983). It can be interrupted by many events, such as meningitis, dehydration, or undernutrition (Gilles, 1983; Gilles, Shankle, & Dooling, 1983; Leviton & Gilles, 1983). Little is known about its robustness given altered sensory inputs.

Concurrent with the processes of cell differentiation, myelination, and neurobehavioral differentiation, neurochemical development occurs. The passage of impulses or messages between cells is accomplished by chemical neurotransmitters, which often are released only if up to four or five different regulatory systems concur in specific configurations. More than two dozen neurotransmitters have so far been identified, and no doubt there are many more. The sensitivities and densities of receptors for certain neurotransmitters vary widely from brain region to region and are very much influenced by experience. The brain and sensory organs are continuously interdependent for structural and functional development. As the complex events and characteristics of brain development outlined above show, it may well be disadvantageous to be born before term because the brain may not be functionally prepared to meet the demands of the extrauterine environment (Gilles, 1983).

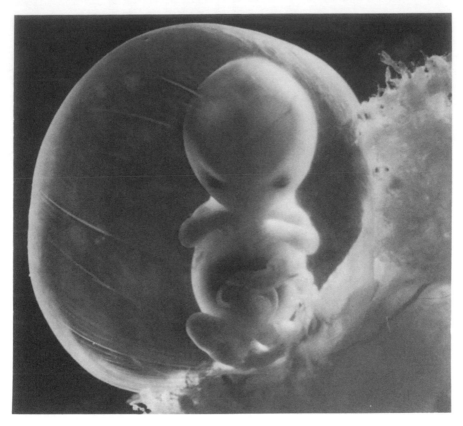

Figure 2.6 Seven weeks old, nearly an inch long, and weighing about two grams: spontaneous exploratory behavior. (Reprinted with permission from Nilsson, 1973)

The vulnerability of support structure tissue adds to the picture of difference in sensitivity and fragility of the preterm brain and the consequent sensitivity in an infant's overall functional modulation. At 24–28 weeks, having supported the massive cortical cell generation, the germinal matrix is still highly vascular (Volpe, 1995). With active neuronal migration away from germinal matrix, the tissue becomes susceptible to hemorrhage. Up to 50% of preterms born before 32 weeks have some degree of hemorrhage and the incidence increases with the reduction in gestational age (Volpe, 1995).

Given the further elaboration of the cortex from the 28th to the 40th week of fetal life, it is not surprising that the impact on CNS organization of unexpected experiences may be significant. Animal models have provided substantial evidence that specific environmental inputs are necessary for support of normal cortical ontogenesis in the course of sensitive periods of brain development (Duffy, Burchfiel, & Snodgrass, 1978; Duffy et al., 1984; Mower, Burchfiel, & Duffy, 1982; Spinelli, Jensen, & DePrisco, 1980). When the expected environmental inputs are not forthcoming, the involved mechanisms actively inhibit developing pathways through overactivation of existing functional pathways. These mechanisms are inferred from, for instance, the successful experimental reactivation by gamma-aminobutyriz acid (GABA) and morphine antagonists of functionally suppressed neurons located in the visual cortex (Duffy et al., 1984.) The hypothesis is particularly appealing, given the hierarchical ordering of endorphin receptor sites in primates. With the substantial increase in the evolutionarily more recent, and ontogenetically later association cortical areas, culminating in frontal cortex (Lewis et al., 1981), it is not surprising that the preterm infant is at increased risk for developmental difficulties in these domains (Als, 1995; Duffy et al., 1990). The frontal lobe is the area strongly implicated in attention, learning, and executive function deficit in the school-age population (Denckla, 1993).

Further support for such a brain-based formulation of understanding preterm functioning comes from the Goldman-Rakic research team, which has shown that the specific connection systems developed in primates involve not only competition between axon terminals and trophic feedback between pre-and postsynaptic cells but also dynamic modification of connections at long distances by functional activity (Easter, Purves, Rakic, & Spitzer, 1985; Rakic, 1988). They conclude that changes in activity of distant yet synaptically related structures that reduce or change specific input to the cortex will affect subsequent developmental events and provide the setting for new cell relations, the net outcome of which appears to be the emergence of unique cerebral cyto-and chemoarchitectonic maps (Rakic, 1991; Rakic, Suñer, & Williams, 1991). Changes induced in midgestation in monkey thalamic fiber projections have yielded the formation of a hybrid cortex, indicating that during rapid brain development new cytoarchitectonic regions may arise depending on the unique combinations of intrinsic properties of the cortical neurons and afferent fibers involved (Rakic et al., 1991).

Not only thalamic changes appear to have profound effects on cortical organization but differential cell death of up to 50% of neurons in layers II–IV (Heuman & Leuba, 1983), and other events of differential axon retraction in the cortical plate itself, which begin around 24 weeks gestation with the decrease of cell migration, appear to be of key importance in sculpting the developing cortex (Finlay & Miller, 1993). These normally occurring events take place at a time when the condition of prematurity can have an adverse effect on brain development (Finlay & Miller, 1993). The documentation of cortical heterotopias (abnormally placed tissue) in the brains of some learning disabled individuals (Galaburda & Kemper, 1979; Rosen, Sherman, & Galaburda, 1993) and the more recent evidence of last-trimester leptomeningeal heterotopias (abnormally placed tissue on the lining of the brain), which in turn lead to secondary cortical alterations (Marin-Padilla, 1993), document the likely difference in brain and behavioral function of prematurely born infants. These phenomena also lead one to consider the nature of the process of cortical cell migration and cell death itself as much more dynamic than previously assumed.

Germinal matrix volume, as shown in Figure 2.7 (Gilles et al., 1983a and b), has reached its peak at 23–25 weeks. Monoclonally organized cells in the ger-

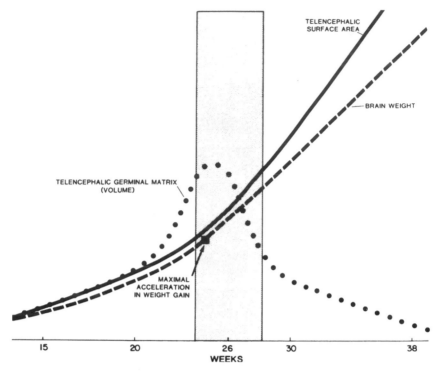

Figure 2.7 At the end of the second trimester (shaded bar) there is a marked change in brain weight with maximal rate acceleration at 24.5 weeks. At the end of gestation the rate of brain growth is maximal. Telencephalic surface area growth is similar. The absolute volume of the telencephalic germinal matrix reaches a maximum at the end of the second trimester, then rapidly declines. (Reprinted with permission from Gilles, 1983)

minal matrix, in contrast to previous evidence (Rakic, 1988), do not necessarily migrate together and may end up in quite divergent regions (Walsh & Cepko, 1992), suggesting complex communication between cells during the migratory process. Of great interest is the more recent research on the function of subplate neurons (De Carlos & O'Leary, 1992; Ghosh & Shatz, 1993; McConnell, Ghosh & Shatz, 1989). These neurons arise in the generative zones and migrate to the primitive marginal zone before generation and migration of the neurons of the cortical plate occurs (Volpe, 1995). The apparent function of the subplate neurons (De Carlos & O'Leary, 1992; Ghosh & Shatz, 1993; McConnell et al., 1989) appears to be to provide a site for synaptic contact for axons ascending from the thalamus and other cortical sites. These axons are termed "waiting" thalamo-cortical and cortico-cortical afferents, because their neuronal targets in the cortical plate have not yet arrived or differentiated. These subplate neurons have been shown to establish a functional synaptic link between waiting afferents and their cortical targets and also appear to guide ascending axons to their targets. When subplate neurons are experimentally eliminated, thalamo-cortical afferents destined for the overlying cortex fail to move into the cortex and continue to grow aimlessly in the subcortical region (Volpe, 1995). Thus, subplate neurons appear to be strongly involved in cerebral cortical organization. Furthermore, their descending axon collaterals appear to guide the initial projections from cerebral cortex toward subcortical and other cortical sites. The subplate neuron layer in the human frontal cortex reaches its peak as late as 22–34 weeks of gestation, a time the preterm infant spends outside of the womb. These areas include the visual cortex, which in the womb would receive no light or pattern input, and the auditory cortex, which in the womb receives stimuli of a kind quite different from that outside the womb.

It seems likely that messages transmitted from these primary cortical regions to other cortical areas, including the prefrontal cortex, are different for the preterm than they would be for the fetus. Programmed cell death appears to begin generally late in the third trimester and extends to well after the sixth month postterm in frontal association cortex. Regions such as the somatosensory and visual cortices appear to have only slightly different time courses. Consequently, the timing and pattern of cell death and selective elimination of neuronal processes and synapses appear to critically influence brain organization (Allsopp, 1993; Catsicas, Thanos, & Clarke, 1987; Driscoll & Chalfie, 1992; Ferrer, Soriano, & Delrio, 1992; Oppenheim, 1991; Oppenheim, Schwartz, & Shatz, 1992; Purves & Lichtman, 1980).

The loss of neurons may serve two major developmental functions. First, the loss may adjust interconnecting populations of neurons by eliminating aberrant projections. It may refine synaptic connections and correct presumed errors, thereby sculpting pathways unique to the individual. Second, it may serve in the removal of terminal axonal branches and their synapses. Likely, these differentiating events are modified when the brain is injured or finds itself in unusual sensory circumstances, as is the case for the prematurely born infant, and cells might be preserved that otherwise would be eliminated and vice versa. Supporting evidence comes from monkeys delivered experimentally prematurely. While unchanged in visual cortical cell number, they showed significantly different cortical synapse formations with respect to cell size, cell type, and laminar distribution. These differences correlated with the degree of prematurity when compared to full-term monkeys tested at comparable postterm ages (Bourgeois, Jastreboff, & Rakic, 1989).

Thus, while some events may influence neuronal migration per se (Rakic, 1990), other events, including differences in sensory input, may alter cortico-cortical connections, thereby leading to unique cyto-and chemoarchitectures of the cerebral cortex. This supports the hypothesis that preterm infants are likely to show brainbased differences in neurofunctional performance. Premature activation of cortical pathways may inhibit later differentiations and interfere with the appropriate development of the brain, especially for prefrontal connecting systems involved in complex mental processing, attention, and self-regulation (Cornell & Gottfried, 1976; Duffy et al., 1990; Duffy et al., 1984; Linn et al., 1985; Turkewitz & Kenney, 1985).

THE NICU ENVIRONMENT AND BRAIN DEVELOPMENT

In a full-term child, axonal and dendritic proliferation, and the massive increase in outer layer cortical cell growth and differentiation leading to the enormous gyri and sulci formation of the human brain (Cowan, 1979), occurs in mother-mediated protection from environmental perturbations. A steady supply of nutrients, temperature control, and the multiple regulating systems, including those of chronobiological rhythms, are afforded by the intrauterine environment (Reppert & Rivkees, 1989). For the preterm infant, these mechanisms are replaced by stimuli from a very differently organized NICU environment. There is increasing evidence that the NICU environment involves sensory overload and stands in stark sensory mismatch to the developing nervous system's growth requirements (Freud, 1991; Gottfried & Gaiter, 1985; Wolke, 1987). It has been shown that prolonged diffuse sleep states, unattended crying (Hansen & Okken, 1979; Martin, Okken, & Rubin, 1979), supine positioning (Martin, Herrell et al., 1979), routine and excessive handling (Danford et al., 1983; Long, Philip, & Lucey, 1980; Murdoch & Darlow, 1984; Norris, Campbell, & Brenkert, 1982), ambient sound (Long, Lucey, & Philip, 1980), lack of opportunity for sucking (Anderson, Burroughs, & Measel, 1983; Burroughs et al., 1978; Field et al., 1982), and poorly timed social and caregiving interactions (Gorski, et al., 1983) have adverse developmental effects. How does one estimate the potential effects on an infant's nervous system when it moves from the relative equilibrium of the intrauterine aquatic environment to the extrauterine terrestrial environment of the NICU (Alberts & Cramer, 1988)? How does one identify and foster a fetal infant's own strengths in doing so? How does one identify an infant's current vulnerabilities in the mismatch of the brain's expectation and the input from the environment?

DEVELOPMENTAL THEORY AND CONCEPTUAL FRAMEWORK

The principle of phylogenetic and ontogenetic adaptedness concerns the individual organism as an evolving member of a species. The ethologist's construct of adaptedness (Babson, 1970; Blurton Jones, 1972, 1974, 1976) suggests that each organism at any stage of development is evolved to implement not only a species-appropriate but also a species-parsimonious level of adaptedness to its particular niche. Since the process of selection takes place at the level of behavior over generations, many essentials of a species' repertoire may become hardwired, as experimental animal and human studies have documented (Lettvin et al., 1959). In the course of a species' evolution, a surprisingly specific and effective organism-environment fit is ensured at the level of the organism's CNS. The more primitive and simple the organism's nervous system, the more behavioral configurations, or sequences, are likely to be hardwired on a simpler level. The more complex the organism and the more complex and flexible the behavioral interconnections necessary to ensure species survival, the larger the association cortex in comparison to the primary sensory cortex. Softwiring is also more likely and allows for flexibility and complexity of response backed up by a system of multiple checks and balances. The more complex and flexible the organism, the larger the buffering plasticity and organismic *Spielraum*, the idling or play space.

Ethological studies of the interaction between newborn and caregiver have identified, from the prenatal period on, the importance, complexity, and subtlety of the parent-infant interactions. While the human newborn shares in the ventro-ventral primate *Tragling* (being carried) configuration (Hassenstein, 1973), the human newborn depends on the parents' active physical support for successful carrying.

Positive elicitors, which emotionally fuel the caregiver, are not only available but, it appears, are required early on to keep parents socially and affectively close to human infants, who are motorically ineffectual in assuring closeness to the parent necessary for their survival. Immediately after birth the connections between the newborn's eye opening and visual attention and his or her parent's affectionate behavior demonstrate a complex homeostatic regulation (Als, 1975, 1977; Grossman, 1978; Minde et al., 1980; Robson, 1967). These behaviors appear to function as mutual releasers launching both partners on their path of complex affective and cognitive interchange, fueling mutual competence well beyond discomfort removal, caretaking, and feeding. The ethologist's principle of adaptedness thus sharpens one's observations in seriously considering all of an organism's behavior at each stage of species adaptation. It further identifies a human newborn as a socially competent and active partner in a feedback system with a caregiver, seeking and eliciting that physiological, motoric, state, and attentional interactive organization from the environment that the newborn requires to assure self-actualization. The evolutionary importance of this earliest extrauterine social-affective connection is revealed by the simultaneous evolutionary differentiation of facial musculature, highlighting the species-specific facial repertoire of the human, which supports subtle, complex, and flexible facial expression from birth on (Fig. 2.8). This repertoire of behaviors (reflects) the highly differentiated, complex, and flexible social nature and structure of humans, which is the postulated species adaptation that assures species survival (Als, 1982a). Comparative studies of facial displays in other primates strengthen the hypothesis that human newborn behaviors, especially facial behaviors, have evolutionary significance. Buettner-Janusch (Buettner-Janusch, 1966) observed throughout the order Primates a correlation between the degree of complexity of social group and the degree of facial flexibility. Bolwig (Bolwig, 1959a, 1959b, 1964) and Andrew (Andrew, 1963a, 1963b), following the earlier work of Huber (1931), also stress the enormous change in facial morphology and behavior observable when one compares the solitary, largely nocturnal prosimian (Figure 2.8A) to the increasingly flexible social diurnal monkey (Fig. 2.8B), ape (Fig. 2.8C), and human (Fig. 2.8D). Aside from the decreasing importance of the overriding platysma muscle and the increasing differentiation of the musculature around the eyes and in the lower face, some morphological features in humans go beyond the facial communication repertoire even of the great apes: the everted red lips emphasizing the line of the mouth, the large area of the eyeball

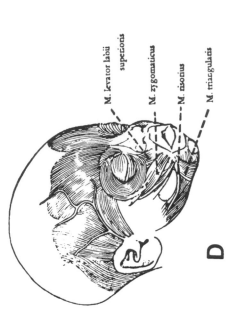

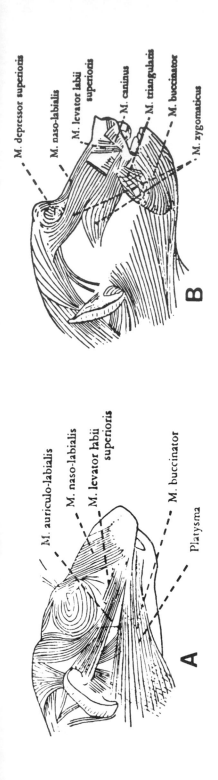

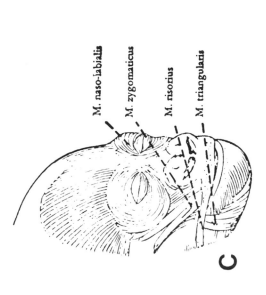

Figure 2.8 A. Lemur; B. Catarrhine Monkey, Papio; C. Gorilla; D. Human Child (Reprinted with permission from Bolwig, 1964)

visible around the pigmented iris, and the increased muscular independence of the periocular and perioral muscles groups. This suggests that from birth on, human newborns are structured to actively elicit the emotional and affective/cognitive support and input that furthers their own increasing behavioral differentiation and organization (Als, 1977). Human newborns are active shapers of their own development, and their interactive attentional capacity seems paramount, in keeping with their species-specific humanness.

The application of the principles of organism-environment transaction to the study of the human newborn (Sander, 1962, 1964, 1970, 1976, 1980) has identified the interplay of various subsystems of functioning within the organism. These systems influence an infant's physiological functioning, motor activity, and state organization as they interact with the caregiving environment. The adaptive task for the infant is to achieve phase synchrony between periodicities that characterize these different systems, as well as synchronization between internal events and the environment (Sander, 1975, 1980; Sander et al., 1979). Poorly timed stimuli penetrate and disrupt all subsystems, while appropriately timed stimuli appear to maintain and enhance functional integration and support growth. Caregivers need to identify synchronous, cohesive functioning and the thresholds to disruption.

According to Denny-Brown (1962, 1966), a motor system physiologist, underlying the organism's evolving toward smooth integration is the tension between two basic antagonists of behavior, as seen in movement disorders such as athetosis. There are two basic physiological types of responses, namely, the exploratory and the avoiding response, the toward and the away, the approaching or reaching out, and the withdrawing or defending response. The two responses at times are released together and conflict with one another. If a threshold of organization-appropriate stimulation is passed, one may abruptly switch into the other. Proof for the basic nature of these two poles of behavior includes single cells in the somatosensory cortex programmed to produce total body-toward movements upon stimulation and other single cells programmed to produce total body-avoidance movements (Duffy & Burchfiel, 1971). The same basic principle has been shown to operate in the process of the gradual specialization of central arousal processes leading to functionally adaptive patterns, such as suckling, nipple-grasping, huddling, and others, for instance, in altricial animals (Rosenblatt, 1976; Schneirla, 1959, 1965; Schneirla & Rosenblatt, 1961, 1963).

The principles outlined here are thought to be relevant to fetal infants, who enter the extrauterine environment too early. The principle of dual antagonist integration is helpful in understanding the behavioral patterns of preterm infants to assess thresholds from integration to disorganization. In the integrated performance, the toward and away antagonists modulate each other in an adaptive response. If an input is compelling to an infant and stimulates its interest and internal readiness, it will approach the input, react and interact with it, seek it out, and become sensitized to it. If the input exceeds the infant's capacity to respond, it will actively avoid the input and withdraw from it. Both responses mutually modulate each other. For instance, a full-term newborn is drawn to the animated face of the interacting caregiver. As the attention intensifies, its eyes widen, eyebrows rise, and mouth shapes toward the interactor (Als, 1975, 1977). If the dampening mechanisms of this intensity are not established, as in the immature or preterm infant, the whole head may move forward, arms and legs may thrust toward the interactor, and fingers and toes will extend toward the stimulus. Early on, the response involves the entire body in an undifferentiated way and gradually will become confined largely to the face (Als, Lester, & Brazelton, 1979). The differentiation process appears to be regulated through such homeostatic infant behaviors as averting the eyes, yawning, sneezing, or hiccuping, or it may be regulated by the caregiver through kissing, nuzzling, or moving the infant closer, thus resetting the cycle (Als. 1975, 1977). If neither of these regulation mechanisms is brought into play, or if the initial input is too strong, the infant may turn away, grimace, extend his arms to the side, arch his trunk, splay his fingers and toes, cry, hiccup, spit up, stop breathing, or defecate. In short, the infant will engage in avoidance behaviors at various levels of functioning. Thus, very early behavioral functioning may be conceptualized as the continual negotiation of a fetal infant's develop (Als, 1978, 1979, 1982b, 1982c, 1983; Brazelton & Als, 1979).

The initial overriding issue for a premature newborn appears to be the stabilization and integration of physiological functions, such as respiration, heart rate, temperature control, digestive function, and elimination, for which the infant typically requires medical technological support, such as the respirator, incubator, intravenous feeding, and so forth. A premature infant's competent motor system at the corresponding fetal stage is capable of initiating and maintaining flexion, rotation, hand to mouth motion, sucking, grasping, and so on.

State organization and other periodicities, no longer supported by the maternal sleep-wake and rest-activity cycles, or by the maternal hormonal and nutritional cycles, are now influenced by the rhythm of the NICU environment. Thus, a model of synactive subsystem differentiation emerges (Als, 1982b), which highlights the simultaneity of all subsystems in their interaction with one another and with the environment. In this model, the entire system continually reopens and progresses to a new level of more differentiated integration, from which, in turn, the next emerging subsystem differentiation occurs, progressing to more sophisticated and integrated levels of physiological and behavioral organization throughout the life span (Als, 1979, 1982b, 1982c, 1983; Als et al., 1982a, 1982b). To paraphrase Erikson (1962), self-actualization is participation with the world and interaction with another with a "minimum of defensive maneuvers and a maximum of activation, a minimum of idiosyncratic distortion and a maximum of joint validation."

THE BEHAVIORAL LANGUAGE OF THE PRETERM INFANT

In this model one can estimate, by observing an infant's behavior the expectation of the fetal brain for input and the developmental goals of the infant for coregulatory support. This approach postulates that an infant's own behavior provides the best information base from which to estimate its current capabilities and to infer what the infant attempts to accomplish and what processes lead to each level of differentiation. On the basis of this information, one can estimate which supports might further an infant's competencies and shore up overall neurobehavioral organization, even in the face of necessary medical and nursing procedures. Because an infant is seen as continuously and actively self-constructing (Fischer & Rose, 1994), the task of care becomes one of collaboration with the infant. Support for a premature infant combines knowledge of the fetal brain with knowledge of behavioral developmental progression. The developmental functioning of the full-term infant provides a biological blueprint, yet for the preterm infant, it is modified by the altered environment-fetus transaction and by each infant's individual characteristics and needs. By accurately interpreting an infant's behavior, one can construct an appropriate caregiving environment (Als, 1982b).

Even the earliest, most fragile infants display autonomic and visceral responses such as respiration patterns, color fluctuations, spitting, gagging, hiccuping and straining. Other typical behaviors include movement patterns, postures, trunkal tone and the tone of extremities and face, reflected as finger splaying, arching, and grimacing, among others. One can easily observe these signs, as well as levels of awakeness, or states, such as sleeping, wakefulness, aroused upset, and their characteristics (Als, 1983, 1984; Als et al., 1982a).

An infant's behavioral repertoire thus far has been identified through three main subsystems: the autonomic, the motor, and the state. An infant's communication with the environment along these subsystem lines is readily accessible for observation even without instrumentation and indicates whether current circumstances support an infant's functioning or tax it (Als, 1982b; Als et al., 1986). Infant behavior can be understood as involving these basic subsystems, presented in Table 2.1.

The autonomic system's functioning is observable in an infant's breathing patterns, color fluctuation, and visceral stability or instability. Examples of the autonomic system's responses include respiratory regularities or irregularities, skin changes such as cyanosis or pallor, and visceral stability reflected in, for instance, hiccuping, gagging, or spitting up.

Motor system integrity and functioning are assessed by observing an infant's body tone, postural repertoire, and movement patterns, as reflected in facial and trunkal tone, tone of the extremities and in the extensor and flexor postures and movements of face, trunk, and limbs.

State organization is observable in an infant's range of available states, their robustness and modulation, and the patterns of transition from state to state. Some infants show the full continuum of states from deep sleep to light sleep,

Table 2.1. Behavioral Systems and Channels of Communication

	Systems		
	Autonomic	Motor	State
Channels of Communication	Respiration pattern	Tone	Range of states
	Color	Postural repertoire	Robustness of states
	Visceral stability	Movements	Transition patterns

then to drowsy and quiet alert, to active awake and aroused, and then to upset and crying (Brazelton, 1973). Other infants during interactions move from sleep to aroused states and immediately back to sleep again, skipping the alert state. In short, state stability and the smooth transition from state to state reflect intact state organization and CNS control whereas the opposite would reflect CNS disorganization.

To document an infant's communication, a behavior observation sheet has been developed for the recording of detailed observations of an infant's naturally occurring behaviors in the NICU. This continuous time sampling method uses 2-minute recording intervals. Figure 2.9 shows the sheet, designed to be used by trained observers at the infant's bed or care site. The observer does not interact directly with an infant but stands close by, watching it. In order to understand the infant's current functioning and thresholds of stability of the autonomic, motor, and state organizational systems, observation usually lasts at least 60–90 minutes. This includes about 10 minutes of observation before a caregiving interaction with the infant, during the caregiving interaction (e.g., vital sign taking, suctioning, diaper changing, and feeding), and about 10 minutes following the caregiving interaction. Such an observation, especially if repeated at least weekly, yields specific information regarding an infant's robustness and development (Als, 1981; Als et al., 1986, 1994). The observations may then form the basis for caregiving suggestions and modifications in environmental structuring, as discuss later.

The materials necessary for an observation are enough observation sheets to afford a full record of an infant's behavior (one for every 10 minutes) a separate form to collect documentation of the infant's medical history and current status, a quiet pen or pencil, a timepiece with an easily visible second hand, and a clipboard to hold the recording sheets. Depending on the specific purpose of the observation, and to avoid bias, it may be helpful to obtain the infant's history after rather than before an observation. An estimation of an infant's history based on its behavioral picture sharpens one's understanding of the issues it may confront, especially when the behavioral picture and recorded history differ. Appendix A shows the history-recording sheet as part of the example provided. The observation sheet is set up as a frequency checklist for continuous recording of behavior segmented into 2-minute intervals. It does not permit the accurate documentation of duration of a behavior within each 2-minute interval. However, detail on predominant or incidental occurrences within the 2-minute block is accurate enough for the reconstruction of the child's behavioral picture. In the top left row of the sheet, the starting time of the observation is marked; below it are 2-minute time blocks across the page. Each page accommodates 10 minutes of observation time, in five 2-minute columns.

In addition to the recording of detailed behaviors, the lower right-hand section of the page accommodates the recording of an infant's specific location and position, the current caregiving events (manipulations), and sampling of an infant's heart rate (HR), respiratory rate (RR), and pulse oximeter or transcutaneous oxygen monitor readings (TcPO$_2$). Respirations are counted for the first 30 seconds of each 2-minute period, multiplied by two for the recorded respi-

OBSERVATION SHEET Name: _____ Date: _____ Sheet Number _____

		Time:	0-2	3-4	5-6	7-8	9-10
Resp:	Regular						
	Irregular						
	Slow						
	Fast						
	Pause						
Color:	Jaundice						
	Pink						
	Pale						
	Webb						
	Red						
	Dusky						
	Blue						
	Tremor						
	Startle						
	Twitch Face						
	Twitch Body						
	Twitch Extremities						
Visceral/ Resp:	Spit up						
	Gag						
	Burp						
	Hiccough						
	BM Grunt						
	Sounds						
	Sigh						
	Gasp						
Motor:	Flaccid Arm(s)						
	Flaccid leg(s)						
	Flexed/Tucked Arms Act. Post.						
	Flexed/Tucked Legs Act. Post.						
	Extend Arms Act. Post.						
	Extend Legs Act. Post.						
	Smooth Mvmt Arms						
	Smooth Mvmt Legs						
	Smooth Mvmt Trunk						
	Stretch/Drown						
	Diffuse Squirm						
	Arch						
	Tuck Trunk						
	Leg Brace						
Face:	Tongue Extension						
	Hand on Face						
	Gape Face						
	Grimace						
	Smile						

		Time:	0-2	3-4	5-6	7-8	9-10
State:	1A						
	1B						
	2A						
	2B						
	3A						
	3B						
	4A						
	4B						
	5A						
	5B						
	6A						
	6B						
	AA						
Face (cont.):	Mouthing						
	Suck Search						
	Sucking						
Extrem.:	Finger Splay						
	Airplane						
	Salute						
	Sitting On Air						
	Hand Clasp						
	Foot Clasp						
	Hand to Mouth						
	Grasping						
	Holding On						
	Fisting						
Attention:	Fuss						
	Yawn						
	Sneeze						
	Face Open						
	Eye Floating						
	Avert						
	Frown						
	Ooh Face						
	Locking						
	Cooing						
	Speech Mvmt.						
Posture:	(Prone, Supine, Side)						
Head:	(Right, Left, Middle)						
Location:	(Crib, Isolette, Held)						
Manipulation:							
	Heart Rate						
	Respiration Rate						
	TcPO$_2$						

(vertical text at right margin: 2002 02 1M (12/83))

Figure 2.9 Sample observation sheet. (Reprinted with permission from Als et al., 1986)

ratory rate; HR and TcPO$_2$, or oxygen saturation, readings are recorded from the respective monitors. Actual counting of respirations documents the relative stability and other characteristics of an infant's respirations, which are described in the upper left-hand block of the recording sheet. Color appears below on the left, followed by additional autonomic system behaviors, such as tremors, startles, and twitches, and other specific visceral and respiratory behaviors. Specific motor system behaviors on the left include characteristics of tone, flexor and/or extension postures, arm and leg movements, specific limb and trunk behaviors such as squirming or arching, and facial gestures such as limp, open mouth gestures (gape face), grimacing, smiling, and mouthing. Specific postures and movements of arms, hands, fingers, legs, feet, and toes appear in the right column. State-related behaviors are grouped with the actual states themselves, which are characterized as either robust (B states) or diffuse (A states). Specific state-related behaviors include fussing, yawning, frowning, and so on. Appendix B gives the definitions of each of the behaviors (Als, 1981).

In a descriptive narrative, an infant's environment is first described in terms of light, sound, and activity (see Appendix A). The behavioral picture derived from the observation period preceding the caregiving interaction is then described, in its relationship to HR, RR, and blood oxygen levels. Then, the caregiving interaction and its effect on the infant is documented, with specific behaviors observed again in relation to HR, RR, and oxygen levels. The infant's efforts to integrate the effects of the interaction and the caregiver's efforts to aid the infant are described. As pointed out, the infant uses strategies and mechanisms to move away from and avoid inappropriate environmental demands or configurations or to seek out and move toward inputs currently appropriate for the infant's intake capacities. Avoidance behaviors are believed to reflect stress. Approach and self-regulation behaviors may shift and become stress behaviors, and, similarly, stress behaviors, when successful in reducing stress, may become self-regulatory strategies. In this model, extension behaviors primarily are thought to reflect stress, and flexion behaviors are thought to reflect self-regulatory competence. Diffuse behaviors are thought to reflect stress and well-defined robust behaviors reflect self-regulatory balance. Thus, *self-regulatory balance* is reflected in, for instance, regular smooth respirations, which are neither too fast nor too slow and are not interspersed with pauses. Other evidence of this balance is pink color; no tremors, startles, and twitches; no visceral signs; no flaccidity, smooth, but not overly flexed active tone and arm, leg, and trunkal position; smooth movements of arms, legs, and trunk; and efforts and successes at tucking trunk and limbs together. These characteristics represent effective self-regulation: suck-searching and sucking; hand and foot clasping; hand-to-mouth efforts; grasping and holding on; robust states; raising of eyebrows (face opening); frowning; forward shaping of the mouth (ooh face); looking, cooing, and speech movements; HR between 120 and 160 bpm; RR between 40 and 60 respirations/min; and oxygen saturation, using a pulse oximeter, between 92% and 98%. *Stress and a low threshold to react, reflecting great sensitivity*, would be reflected by irregular respirations, overly slow or fast respirations, respiratory pauses, and color other than pink (i.e., pale, mottled, red, dusky, or blue). Other evidence for stress includes tremors, startles, and twitches and visceral signs such as spitting up, gags, hiccups, grunting and bowel movement straining, sounds, gasps, and sighs. Motor signs of stress include flaccidity of the face, arms, legs, and trunk; frequent extensor movements of the arms and legs; stretching and drowning-like behavior; frequent squirming; arching; frequent tongue extensions; grimacing; specific finger, arm, and leg extensions (splaying, airplaning, saluting, sitting on air); frequent fisting; fussing; yawning; sneezing; floating eye movements; and visual averting. Other signs of potential stress are a HR less than 120 bpm or greater than 160; RR of less than 40 or greater than 60 respirations/min; and blood oxygenation of less than 92% or higher than 98%. From such a description a picture emerges about the level of support or relative vigor of sensory input at which the infant moves from self-regulatory balance to stress. Appendix A provides a sample behavior record with descriptions written in a language understandable to parents as well as professionals. The record's purpose is to educate and support the caregivers in understanding the infant's behavioral functioning and seeing the infant as an active structurer and participant in his or her own development.

THE MEANING AND INTERPRETATION OF BEHAVIOR

The behavioral description of an infant's functioning in the course of the observed interaction is anchored in its medical and family history and current medical status. Together, they are the empirical bases from which to estimate an infant's own current developmental goals. The most important question is, what are the infant's physiological and behavioral efforts and needs, not what has the professional caregiver planned next for the infant. For instance, an infant may seek to bring his or her hand and fingers to the mouth in order to suck or may make repeated efforts to breathe smoothly *with* rather than against the respirator, only to be repeatedly interrupted by the fixed respirator settings. The infant may attempt to settle back into sleep and restfulness after being cared for, only to be startled and repeatedly reawakened by sounds from alarms, faucets, voices, or equipment being moved about.

The next step is to respond to the individual infant's expectations concerning the environment and the delivery of care itself. Presumably this will enhance an infant's well-being, sense of competence, effectiveness, and development.

An infant's care involves many procedures, examinations, and therapeutic interventions delivered by staff from various disciplines. Consequently, there is an increased risk for miscommunication between infant and parents and the infant's other caregivers. Primary nursing care is of key importance, for it provides consistency of staffing and continuity in care, thereby fostering an intimate knowledge of infant and family. An infant's communications, as a basis for individualized care delivery, are much more effectively utilized in care planning and care delivery in a primary care model than in traditionally scheduled staffing models. Primary care, in this context, involves a primary nursing team, as well as a primary physician, respiratory therapist, social worker, physical or occupational therapists, and primary representatives from other disciplines as indicated. In such a model, parents are active members of the primary team and participate in rounds, care conferences, decision making, and care implementation.

Experience in developmental care practice has shown that developmentally trained professionals are of key importance in helping the care teams of specialty disciplines maintain a consistent developmental perspective in their care planning for the infant. Qualifications for such developmental specialists include background and training in infant mental health or developmental and child psychology, with specialization in NICU work. The role of the developmentalist includes, among other responsibilities, review and documentation of an infant's sleep and wake cycles in each 24-hour day to increase the organization of robust sleep and wake cycles. The developmentalist will safeguard the emotional health and well-being of infant and family by assuring continuity and intimacy of primary relationships for the infant. Advocacy for early skin-to-skin holding as soon after admission as possible, parent integration into the caregiving and nurturing of the infant on a consistent basis, successful breast-feeding, and inclusion of other family members all support an infant's and family's emotional well-being and overall functioning. The developmentalist provides formal and consistently scheduled observations, which assist the formulation of individualized primary care plans with suggested input for the specialists in the NICU. The focus of this framework is on an infant's strengths and supports its connection with par-

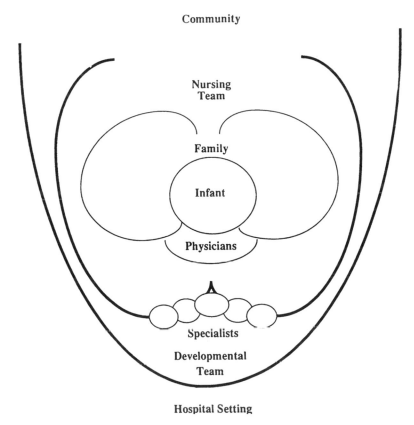

Figure 2.10 Developmental NICU Care Model

ents and family. Finally, the developmental professionals facilitate the invitation of community-based early intervention providers to the NICU so they can meet and learn from infant, family, and NICU staff about the infant's course before transition from the NICU. Figure 2.10 conceptualizes such a developmental synactive model of care delivery, with the focus of care on infant and family. The immediate safeguard of structured care is the primary nursing team in collaboration with primary physician(s), supported by specialists, such as respiratory, occupational, and physical therapists, and social workers. The example provided in Appendix A shows the developmental specialist's recommendations based on the observation of the infant's behavior and intended to aid the staff invested in providing supportive care.

TESTING THE VALIDITY OF AN INDIVIDUALIZED, BEHAVIORALLY BASED DEVELOPMENTAL APPROACH TO NICU CARE

To test the efficacy of the neurodevelopmental approach to care that supports CNS development in the unlesioned brain, Buehler et al. (1995) studied a sample of healthy low-risk preterm infants, free of known focal and suspected lesions. Twenty-four consecutively inborn preterm singleton infants cared for in a 16-bed level II SCN were randomly assigned to an experimental or a control group. They were <34 weeks gestational age at birth, of appropriate weight for gestational age; with uneventful labor and delivery histories. They did not require mechanical ventilation for more than 24 hours, were genetically and neurologically intact, and had healthy mothers. The experimental group infants were formally observed within the first 24 hours after birth and every seventh day thereafter. The group received ongoing individualized developmental care by a developmental psychologist in collaboration with a developmentally trained nurse clinician. Control group infants received the standard of care practiced throughout the SCN. A group of 12 healthy full-term infants was studied as a comparison group. While the preterm experimental group infants showed no differences in terms of medical outcome compared to the preterm control group or the full-term group, significant differences among the three groups appeared on two behavioral outcome measures, the Assessment of Preterm Infants' Behavior (APIB) (Als et al., 1982a, 1982b) and the Prechtl Neurological Evaluation (Prechtl, 1977). Four of the six APIB system scores showed significant group differences (Fig. 2.11). As the post hoc pair-wise comparisons indicate, the preterm group displayed the least well-organized behavioral performance, whereas the preterm experimental and full-term groups were behaviorally comparable. The preterm control group was significantly less well-organized than the preterm experimental group on autonomic, motor, and attentional parameters. The preterm control group also differed significantly from the full-term comparison group on measures of autonomic, motor, and regulatory organization. No significant pair-wise differences were found between the preterm experimental group and the full-term comparison group. For an additional 5 of the 18 standard APIB summary variables tested, significant differences among the three

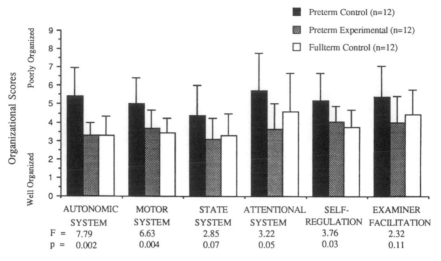

Figure 2.11 Means and standard deviations of the APIB subsystem scores for the preterm control, preterm experimental, and full-term comparison groups derived from the behavioral examination at 2 weeks post expected date of confinement (EDC). Behavioral systems are the autonomic system, the motor system, the state organizational system, the attentional system, the self-regulatory system, and the degree of examiner facilitation necessary in the course of the examination. All system scores are scaled from 1 to 9, with 1 representing well-organized performance and 9 representing poorly organized performance. The six system scores are based on means of 18 scores per system obtained in the course of an examination for each child on the autonomic, motor, state, and self-regulation system; the means of three scores are obtained on the attentional system, and the means of six scores on the variable examiner facilitation. (Reprinted with permission from Buehler et al., 1995)

groups emerged (Fig. 2.12). Again, the preterm control group showed the poorest performance. Each of the four scores showed a consistent orderly progression among the three groups. The preterm control group was the least well-modulated, the preterm experimental group the second best modulated, and the full-term group the most well-modulated.

Measures of electrophysiological function also showed significant improvement for the intervention preterm group compared to the control preterm group. Of a possible total of 180 variables, 70 showed significant differences between the two preterm groups. Nineteen of the 70 resulted from the visual evoked response in alert state (VERA), 12 from the visual evoked response in quiet sleep (VERQ), 13 from the auditory evoked response (AER) to speech (SPE), 14 from AER to nonspeech (NSP), and 12 from AER to click (CLK). Twenty-eight involved the right hemisphere, 24 the left hemisphere, and 18 were bihemispheric. Only nine features were expected to reach significance by chance alone at the <.05 probability level (Maus & Endresen, 1979).

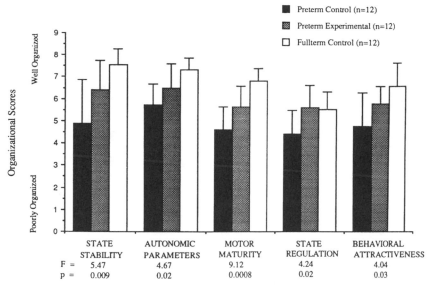

Figure 2.12 Means and standard deviations of the APIB summary scores showing significant differences between the preterm control, preterm experimental, and full-term comparison groups at 2 weeks post-EDC. Summary scores are scaled from 1 to 9, with 1 representing poorly organized performance and 9 representing well-organized performance. State stability measures a combination of parameters, which include lability of states, ability to quiet when motorically aroused, ability to be consoled when motorically aroused, rapidity of build-up to motorical arousal, and degree of discharge smiles versus stimulus-related smiles in alertness. Autonomic parameters include the degree of tremulousness, startles, skin color lability, and the threshold to color change. Motor maturity measures the degree of flaccidity versus hypertonicity and the degree of smoothness and control of limb movements. State regulation consists of the range and flexibility of states, irritability, robustness in handling the examination, control over input, and improvement with facilitation. Behavioral attractiveness measures the overall organization and modulation paired with social responsiveness an engagement. (Reprinted with permission from Buehler et al., 1995)

When all 3 groups were compared, 41 of the 70 features continued to show significant among-group differences. In a large number of these features, 32 of the 41, the preterm experimental group was comparable to the full-term group, while both differed from the preterm control group ($\chi^2 = 34.6$, df = 1, significant at $p \leq .01$). This suggests that the frequency of similarity observed between the full-term and the experimental preterm group is not a chance finding. Figure 2.13 displays the 41 regions showing significant group differences. The area most frequently involved was the frontal lobe, with 18 features. Twelve features involved the temporal region and the remaining 11 the central, occipital, and parietal regions. Of the 41 regions identified, 28 showed significant corre-

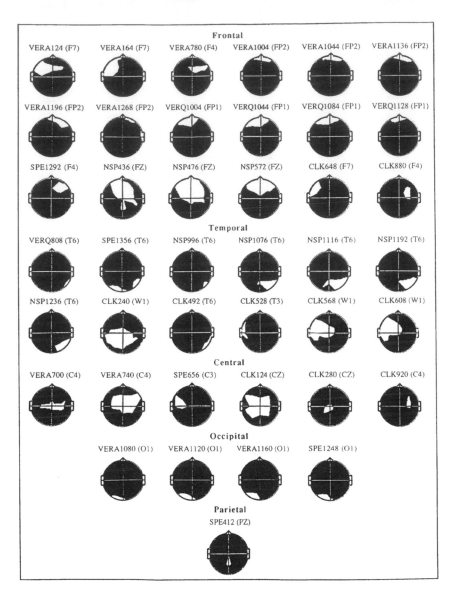

Figure 2.13 Forty-one regions of significant difference ($p \le .05$) among the three groups are shown by qEEG with topographic mapping. Schematic representations are of head areas seen from above (i.e., nose at top, right ear on right side), arranged by locations of regions of difference (ROIs): frontal, temporal, central, occipital, and parietal. Each individual representation indicates the region of difference (white area), evoked potential condition (VERA, VERQ, SPE, NSP, CLK), and starting msec of the 40 msec time period for which a significant between-group difference was identified. The location of the electrode measuring the peak between group difference is in parentheses, identified by region (F = Frontal, FP = Fronto-Polar, T = Temporal, W = Wernicke's, C = Central, O = Occipital, P = Parietal) and side (odd numbers indicate left hemisphere, even numbers right hemisphere, and Z bihemispheric electrode placement). (Reprinted with permission from Buehler et al., 1995)

lations with APIB behavioral measures. The significance ranged from <.05 (83%), to <.01 (16%), to <.001 (1%). Thirteen of these significant correlations were between the frontal lobe features and APIB variables measuring attentional control and state organization. An additional nine features representing the temporal, parietal, and central regions also correlated significantly with APIB measures of attention. The remaining 6 correlations indicated significant relationships with measures of autonomic and motor organization. Thus, the medically healthy preterm infants who received individualized developmental care were more well adjusted autonomically and motorically and especially in terms of state regulation and attentional functioning than the preterm infants who received standard care. Furthermore, they were comparable to the healthy full-term infants with respect to these functions. These neurophysiological differences occurred even though there were no medical differences between the groups at the time of the quantified electroencephalogram (EEG; qEEG) study. The frontal region demonstrated significant correlation with behavioral indices of attentional control and state organization and appeared to show differential vulnerability in the preterm control group. This is not surprising given that, as pointed out earlier, neuronal organization of this region occurs relatively late in the developmental sequence (Huttenlocher, 1984; Schade & van Groenigen, 1961; Yakovlev & Lecours, 1967). Previous studies of prematurity have indicated the frontal region's differential vulnerability (Duffy et al., 1990). It appears that the intervention supports a more full-term differentiation of brain function for these healthy preterm infants and may especially protect frontal lobe functioning.

The individualized developmental approach to environmental support and care based on reading the preterm infant's behavioral cues as described is increasingly advocated for the most high-risk preterm infants also (Becker, Grunwald, Moorman & Stuhr, 1993; Grunwald & Becker, 1990; Lawhon, 1986; Lawhon & Melzar, 1991; VandenBerg, 1990a, 1990b; VandenBerg & Franck, 1990; Wolke, 1987) and has been tested in several studies. Als et al.(1986) found improved medical outcome of VLBW ventilated preterm infants, as evidenced by shorter stays on the respirator, and a decrease in the need for supplemental oxygen and gavage feedings. Improved behavioral outcome at 2 weeks corrected age, as assessed with the APIB (Als et al., 1982a, 1982b) and at 9 months with the Bayley Scale Scores, was also found. Furthermore, there was improved behavioral regulation, as assessed by using a videotaped play paradigm (Kangaroo-Box Paradigm) (Als & Berger, 1986; Als, Duffy, & McAnulty, in press). Becker and others (Becker et al. 1991, 1993; Grunwald & Becker, 1990) found significantly lower scores of morbidity in the first four weeks of hospitalization, as measured with the Minde Daily Morbidity Scale (Minde et al., 1983). There were significantly earlier onset of oral feedings, better average daily weight gain, shorter hospital stays, as well as improved overall behavioral functioning at discharge, as measured with the Neonatal Behavioral Assessment Scale (NBAS) (Brazelton, 1984). Long-term outcome assessed for the Als study (Als et al., 1986) at 18 months and 3 years continues to show a consistent developmental advantage of the experimental group over the control group. The preliminary results from the longitudinal data available from this study show significantly improved

Table 2.2. Medical Outcome Variables*

Variable	Control Group (n = 18)	Experimental Group (n = 20)	df	F	χ^2	p
Average daily weight gain from birth to 2 weeks post-EDC (g)	20 (6)	24 (7)	1, 36	3.18	—	.08
Age post LMP at discharge (wk)	48.3 (17.3)	39.7 (3.1)	1, 18	4.27	—	.05
No. of days in hospital	151 (120)	87 (26)	1, 18	4.78	—	.04
No. of days on mechanical ventilation	63.8 (72.9)	28.3 (23.3)	1, 20	3.93	—	.06
No. of days on oxygen	139.4 (166.1)	56.8 (39.3)	1, 19	4.25	—	.05
No. of days before bottle-feeding	104.1 (85.8)	59.2 (25.8)	1, 18	4.33	—	.05
Pediatric Complication Scale score (mean = 100; SD = 20)	53.1 (2.5)	55.5 (4.4)	1, 31	4.43	—	.04
Hospital charges ($K)	189 (174)	98 (37)	1, 18	4.72	—	.04
Retinopathy of prematurity (ROP)						
None	5	10				
Mild (stages I and II):	10	8				
Moderate (stage III):	3	2				
Severe (stages IV and V):	0	0	2	—	1.99	.37

Bronchopulmonary dysplasia				
None	3	2		
Mild (stage I)	7	13		
Moderate (stage II)	2	5		
Severe (stage III)	6	0		
			—	3	9.21	.03
Pneumothorax				
None	12	19		
Mild	1	1		
Moderate	3	0		
Severe	2	0		
			—	3	6.49	.09
Intraventricular Hemorrhage (IVH)				
None	8	19		
Grade I	3	0		
II	1	0		
III	2	1		
IV	4	0		
			—	4	12.75	.01

*Results are mean $\pm$ SD unless otherwise stated. Brown-Forsythe one-way analysis of variance: F, two tailed; χ^2, two tailed.
EDC = expected date of confinement; LMP = last menstrual period.
Reprinted with permission from Als et al., 1994.

performance of the experimental group at 7 years on a number of the neuro-psychological measures (Als, Duffy, & McAnulty, in preparation).

A further study (Als et al., 1994) has utilized random assignment of infants weighing <1,251 g, born before 30 weeks gestational age, intubated within the first 3 hours after delivery, and requiring mechanical ventilation for at least 24 of the first 48 hours. Eighteen control and 20 experimental group infants met these criteria. For this study, a group of nurses was specially educated and trained in the behaviorally based approach of individualized caregiving. Staffing was structured so that, for the experimental group infants, during at least one shift in every 24-hour cycle, a nurse specially educated in the behavioral approach cared for the infant and family. Formal behavioral observations conducted by a psychologist in collaboration with a developmental clinical nurse specialist began within the first 24 hours and were repeated every tenth day until discharge from the nursery. Again, these observations provided the basis for support to the primary teams for individualization of care for the experimental group infants and their families. Control group infants were identified to the NICU staff within 2 weeks before discharge so as not to influence and bias their staffing and care in any way. The control and experimental groups were comparable on all background variables including birthweight, gestational age at birth, Apgar scores at 1 and 5 minutes, mean and maximum fractions of inspired oxygen (FiO$_2$ in the first 48 hours and the first 10 days, the incidence of patent ductus arteriosus, maternal age, social class, Obstetric Complication Scale Scores (Littman & Parmelee, 1974), gender, ethnicity, birth order, and the use of prenatal corticosteroids. As Table 2.2 indicates, the experimental group infants had shorter hospitalizations, were younger at discharge, had reduced hospital charges, and had improved weight gain to 2 weeks after their due date. They had a reduced rate of IVH and of the severity of chronic lung disease. They also showed improved developmental outcome at 2 weeks corrected age, as measured with the APIB (Als et al., 1982b), with much better functioning in terms of autonomic regulation, motor system performance, and self-regulation (Fig. 2.14). Systematic electrophysiological group differences by qEEG with topographic mapping (Duffy, Burchfiel, & Lombroso, 1979) were also found at 2 weeks postterm, suggesting differences in function in a large central region of the brain, as well as in a large portion of the right occipital hemisphere, in two left parietal, a right parietal, and an additional right occipital region (Fig. 2.15). Two-group stepwise discriminant function analysis, entering all 5 variables numerically representing the regions depicted, yielded a Wilk's Λ of 0.476 ($p <$ .0003), implying a very large difference between the groups. Classification was 83.9% successful.

By 9 months after expected date of confinement (EDC), two infants in the control group were unavailable for study. On assessment with the Bayley Scales of Infant Development, the experimental group, compared to the control group, showed a significantly higher Mental Developmental Index (118.30 $\pm$ 17.35 vs. 94.38 $\pm$ 23.31; F = 12.47; df = 1, 34; p $\leq$ .001) and Psychomotor Developmental Index (100.60 $\pm$ 20.19 vs. 83.56 $\pm$ 17.97; F = 6.97; df = 1,34; p $\leq$ .01).

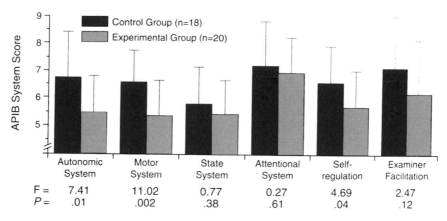

Figure 2.14 Assessment of Preterm Infants' Behavior (APIB) system score 2 weeks after expected date of confinement (mean ± SD). Higher scores represent more poorly organized performance. Score for autonomic, motor, state, and self-regulation are based on 18 scores per infant for the attentional system, three scores, and for the examiner facilitation, six scores. Significant F scores for the autonomic, motor, and self-regulation systems indicate that infants in the experimental group had better functioning of these systems.
(Reprinted with permission from Als et al., 1994)

Furthermore, of 20 infant variables measured in the 6-minute Kangaroo Box Paradigm Play Episode, 16 showed differences favoring the experimental group, in significance range from $<.03$ to $<.0001$. The largest differences were found in gross and fine motor modulation, overflow postures and associated movements, complexity and modulation of combining object and social play, ability to stay engaged in the task, and degree of facilitation necessary to accomplish the task. In the 6-minute Stillface Episode, 12 of 19 infant parameters showed significant group differences (p $<$ .04 to $<$ .0001), again favoring the experimental group infants, (Fig. 2.16 and 2.17). None of the 14 parent variables assessed showed a significant group difference, yet all three interaction variables (turntaking, overall synchrony of the interaction, and overall quality of the interaction variables (p $<$ .0004) favored the experimental group. Thus, the infants in the experimental group appeared significantly more well-organized, well-differentiated, and well-modulated than the control group infants. Canonical correlation between the factors derived from the APIB variables and the factors derived from the K-Box variables was significant (canonical r = .84367; X^2 = 50.77, df = 20, p $<$ .0002). This indicates a strong relationship between overall behavioral regulation at 2 weeks, as measured with the APIB, and overall regulation at 9 months, as measured with the Kangaroo Box Paradigm.

Neither IVH nor BPD had significant indirect effects on any of the medical outcome variables (Table 2.3). In terms of electrophysiological outcome, IVH had a significant indirect effect on only one variable. However, even for this variable the direct intervention effect was stronger. The presence of BPD had

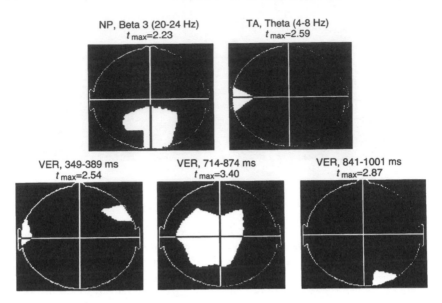

NP, Beta 3 (20-24 Hz)
$t_{max}=2.23$

TA, Theta (4-8 Hz)
$t_{max}=2.59$

VER, 349-389 ms
$t_{max}=2.54$

VER, 714-874 ms
$t_{max}=3.40$

VER, 841-1001 ms
$t_{max}=2.87$

Figure 2.15 Schematic outlines show the nose at the top, the left ear to the left, and the right ear to the right. The white areas represent regions of significant between-group differences ($p < .05$, two-tailed). The state of brain activation and the maximum t value (t_{max}) are as follows: non-processing awake (NP), in the electroencephalographic beta 3 range of 20 to 24 Hz; trace alternant (TA), or quiet sleep, in the electroencephalographic theta range of 4 to 8 Hz; and visual-evoked response (VER) in quiet sleep from the times indicated. There were 14 infants in the control group and 17 in the experimental group.
(Reprinted with permission from Als et al., 1994)

no indirect effect on any of the electrophysiological findings. Neither IVH nor BPD had any significant indirect effects on any of the APIB or Bayley outcome measures. Furthermore, only 2 of the 32 Kangaroo Box measures showed significant indirect IVH effects, namely, symmetry of motor performance in the play and in the stillface episode. None showed indirect BPD effects. Thus, the direct effects of the intervention on outcome appear to go beyond the indirect contribution from reduction in IVH and BPD.

An independent replication study from another center (Fleisher et al., 1995) focused on the same high-risk population and was conducted since the introduction of surfactant in the NICU. The study found significant positive medical and APIB results, although the intervention involved only inservice orientation to the nursing staff and the availability of a developmental professional in support of the experimental group care teams.

In a further study (Als et al., in preparation), the integration of this individualized approach into the NICU was tested by assignment of experimental group high-risk infants to specially trained care teams supported on an ongoing basis by two developmental specialists, who, however, did not conduct serial behavioral observations. Preliminary analysis of outcome again showed reduction in

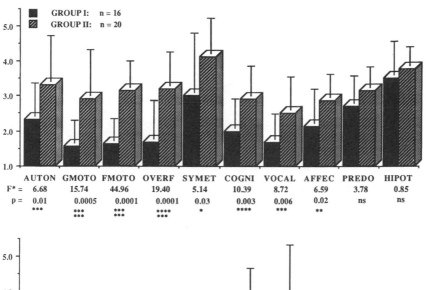

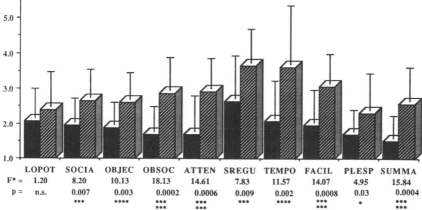

Figure 2.16 Means and standard deviations are presented for 20 parameters of child functioning at 9 months after expected date of confinement (EDC) for the control group (I) and the experimental group (II). The scores are derived from the videotaped observation of child and parent in play (Play Episode) in the Kangaroo Box Paradigm. All variables are behaviorally defined and scaled from 1 to 5; 1 reflects poorly organized performance, 5 reflects well-organized performance. The parameters assessed are autonomic regulation (AUTON); gross motor modulation (GMOTO); fine motor modulation (FMOTO); overflow and associated movements (OVERF); symmetry of motor performance (SYMET); cognitive appreciation of the task (COGNI); vocalization pattern (VOCAL); affective range and regulation (AFFEC); predominant (PREDO), highest (HIPOT) and lowest (LOPOT) affective phase; complexity of interaction with the parent (SOCIA); complexity of interaction with the object (OBJEC); modulation of shifting of attention between parent and object (OBSOC); ability to break the task into manageable components (ATTEN); success in maintaining overall equilibrium in the face of the task (SREGU); modulation of the speed of movements (TEMPO); degree of facilitation needed from the parent (FACIL); degree of pleasure and pride (PLESP); and overall summary rating of competence (SUMMA). Of the 20 variables measured and compared by analysis of variance, using the Brown-Forsythe Equality of Means Test, F^*, which does not assume variances between groups to be equal, 17 showed significant group differences ($p < .05$), favoring the experimental group children. This indicates that the experimental group children performed better than the control group children in terms of behavioral modulation on the majority of parameters measured.

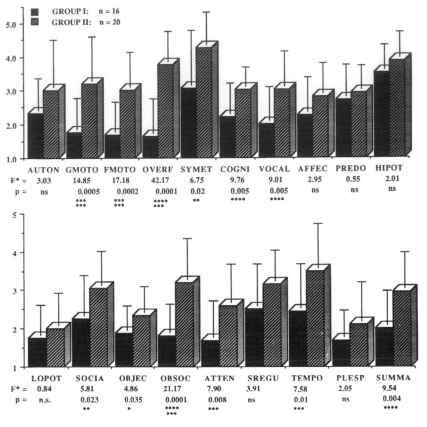

Figure 2.17 Means and standard deviations are presented for 19 parameters of child functioning at 9 months after expected date of confinement (EDC), for the control group (I) and the experimental group (II). The scores are derived from videotaped observation of the child in play with the Kangaroo Box, while the parent is sitting with a still face at the edge of the room, no longer helping the child or interacting with the child in any way (Stillface Episode). All variables are defined as described in Figure 2.16, with the exception of the variable FACIL, which is deleted, and the variable SOCIA, which assesses the child's strategies in eliciting the stillfaced parent's responsiveness. ANOVA, using the Brown-Forsythe Equality of Means Test, F^*, showed 12 of the 19 variables favoring the experimental group infants. Affective organization and self-regulation did not show a significant group difference. Overall, the experimental group was significantly more well-regulated than the control group.

number of days on the ventilator and on gavage tube feedings, decreased length of hospitalization, and improved weight gain, as well as improved developmental outcome at 2 weeks and 9 months after the EDC. There was no decrease in incidence of IVH or severity of chronic lung disease. The IVH effects may well depend on developmental support in the acute first few hours of admission, when systematic feedback may be differentially productive.

Table 2.3. Path Analysis to Medical, Electrophysiological, and Behavioral Outcome Measures via IVH and BPD†

Variable	Direct Effect P_{14}	Indirect Effect IVH $P_{24} \times P_{12}$	Indirect Effect BPD $P_{34} \times P_{13}$	Correlation r
Medical outcome measures (n = 38)				
Age post-LMP at discharge	−0.32*	0.12	−0.14	−0.34*
No. of days in hospital	−0.32*	0.11	−0.15	−0.36*
No. of days on oxygen	−0.31*	0.13	−0.16	−0.34*
No. of days before bottle-feeding	−0.27	0.06	−0.14	−0.35*
Pediatric Complications Scale score	0.24	0.02	0.07	0.32
Hospital charges	−0.27	0.07	−0.16	−0.36*
Electrophysiological Outcome (n = 31)				
Awake nonprocessing, beta3 (20–24 Hz)	0.18	0.23	−0.01	0.41*
Quiet sleep, theta (4–8 Hz)	−0.28	−0.16	0.01	−0.44*
VER from 349–389 msec	0.25	0.19	−0.00	0.44*
VER from 714–874 msec	−0.32*	−0.29*	−0.01	−0.61**
VER from 841–1001 msec	0.15	0.30	−0.00	0.44*
Behavioral Outcome—APIB (n = 38)				
Autonomic system	−0.31*	0.01	−0.12	−0.41*
Motoric system	−0.45*	0.02	−0.05	−0.48***
Self-regulation system	−0.36	0.07	−0.05	−0.34*
Symmetry of orientation	0.53***	−0.02	−0.02	0.49***
Autonomic stability	0.36*	0.00	0.13	0.48***
Modulation of tone, movement, and posture	0.19	0.06	0.10	0.35*
Symmetry of motor performance	0.38	0.03	−0.03	0.39*
Number of abnormal reflexes	−0.50***	0.09	−0.07	−0.49***
Behavioral Outcome—Bayley Scales (n = 36)				
Mental Developmental Index	0.41*	0.04	0.08	0.52***
Psychomotor Developmental Index	0.24	0.07	0.10	0.41*

†The path analysis tests the relationship of the independent variable, namely the experimental treatment, to each of the dependent variables, namely the outcome variables, taking the two intervening variables, intraventricular hemorrhage (IVH) and bronchopulmonary dysplasia (BPD), into account. The direct effect (P_{14}) and the two indirect effects ($P_{24} \times P_{12}$ and $P_{34} \times P_{13}$) sum to yield Pearson product moment correlations (r) between the experimental treatment and the outcome variables. LMP = last menstrual period; VER = visual evoked response; APIB = assessment of preterm infants' behavior.
  *$P\#.05$, two-tailed.
  **$P\#.005$, two-tailed.
  ***$P\#.01$, two-tailed.
  Reprinted with permission from Als et al., 1994.

A current multicenter study involving three different NICUs and using random assignment focuses on ventilator-dependent, very high-risk preterm infants born at ≤ 28 weeks gestation. The study involves inborn as well as transported infants and nurseries employing primary care nursing and conventionally scheduled nursing. Preliminary results appear to validate the effectiveness of the developmental care model in terms of significant improvement, especially in terms of weight gain and growth parameters, and in reduction of length of hospital stay and hospital cost. Developmental outcome, as measured with the APIB, also shows significant improvement. Furthermore, preliminary analysis of the assessment of family functioning shows the experimental group parents were significantly more effective in understanding their infants as individuals and themselves as parents (Als & Gilkerson, 1989–1994).

The studies reviewed involving developmental care for healthy preterm infants and for the very early born, VLBW, and very high-risk preterm infants suggest that differences in experience during the last 16 weeks of gestation differentially influence infants' neurodevelopmental functioning. These differences are measurable at 2 weeks and 9 months postterm and may foreshadow the developmental differences documented for preterm children at preschool and school ages.

THE NIDCAP MODEL: GUIDELINES FOR CARE

The clinical framework of developmental care derived from the conceptual and empirical work outlined has been developed into the Newborn Individualized Developmental Care and Assessment Program (NIDCAP®). This program offers training for professionals in the family-centered individualized approach to care described. To effectively integrate developmentally supportive, family-centered care into NICUs in the NIDCAP® framework, the following guidelines (Holmes, Sheldon & Als, 1995; Vento & Feinberg, in press) have been derived from the experience now available.

Structure the Infant's 24-Hour Day

The primary care team coordinates all interventions across several 24-hour time intervals into individually appropriate clusters timed in accordance with the individual infant's sleep-wake cycles, state of alertness, medical needs, and feeding competence. All interventions are evaluated regarding their necessity and appropriateness for a particular infant. The goal is to provide restfulness and to support growth. Infants' caregiving schedules are coordinated with family schedules to support the integration of the infant into the family and the family into the NICU, and to foster the family's involvement and competence in the child's nurturance and care. During delivery of care, caregivers are expected to approach the infant and family in a calm, attentive manner, explaining to the family the goal and approximate sequence of the care components considered.

Caregivers are encouraged to observe an infant first to understand its current means of communication. They then introduce themselves to the infant using a soft voice and gentle touch, providing periods of rest and recovery between manipulations, containing the infant in a gentle embrace with their hands, or encouraging the parent to do so. Supports such as hands-on containment, sucking on a pacifier or the finger, hand-holding, and hand-to-mouth exploration are ways to encourage dialogue between infant and caregiver and to foster the infant's and the parents' overall competence. During transition periods between caregiving components, caregivers are expected to direct careful attention to the infant's behavior. Typically, increased support is needed as the infant awakens spontaneously, makes efforts to come to alertness, and in turn as the infant returns toward sleep. This is especially the case for very prematurely born infants and those with dysmature or impaired nervous systems, such as infants who experienced birth asphyxia, intrauterine growth retardation, and narcotic or cocaine exposure. Such infants may demonstrate lower thresholds to disorganization. During alert periods caregivers attempt to balance sensory input from the caregiver and from the environment with the infant's current level of alertness and competence. Caregiver interactions are guided by the behavioral cues of the infant toward support of robust wakefulness, increasingly well-focused alertness, and well-modulated social interaction. Furthermore, caregivers are expected to support softly flexed, comfortably aligned positions during sleep, routine care, feeding, bathing, and special procedures. Aids such as blanket rolls, nesting, gentle swaddling, special buntings, and hands-on containment may be helpful. Clothing the infant in soft cotton garments appropriately small in size and covering the infant with a soft cotton or silk blanket have been found to facilitate restfulness and comfort. Physical support is gauged to the infant's competence and is increased or decreased depending on the infant's autonomous maintenance of tone and well-adjusted positions and movements.

Feeding method and frequency are also individualized and based on an infant's competence. The goal is to progress toward infant-initiated and-controlled feeding. To facilitate feeding competence, caregivers decrease environmental stimulation and securely cradle the infant in their arms in semi-upright soft flexion, with hands in midline, free to grasp and hold on, and with legs and feet contained. Feeding success is judged not only by the infant's intake but also by its overall energy levels and autonomic, motor, and state functioning. Feeding is conceptualized as a pleasurable and nurturing experience.

Suction and pulmonary care are performed only when clinically indicated, never on a preset schedule, and always by a two-person team. Routine suctioning of the premature infant and chest physical therapy have been shown to lead to abrupt changes in blood flow velocity, associated with IVH and cerebral infarction and should therefore be avoided (see Chapter 1, this volume). When executed gently, support by the second caregiver, whenever possible the parent, helps contain and stabilize the infant throughout the procedure, thereby lessening potential risks and increasing support to the infant.

Opportunities for skin-to-skin holding and nesting are expected to be available at all times and to all families of NICU infants, including ventilated infants. Reclining chaise longues with foot and head rests and large enough to accommodate two parents should be available at each bedside. Staff are expected to be specially trained in the care and comfort of postpartum parents and of infants for the provision of skin-to-skin nurturing. The parent's body has been found to provide warmth and maintain an infant's stable body temperature. Such physical contact appears to result in more restful sleep in the infant and a sense of calm and fulfillment in the parent. The infant has been found to experience increased respiratory stability with decreased incidence of apnea and bradycardia. Mothers who hold their infant skin-to-skin experience increased milk production as well as success and enjoyment in breast-feeding (see Chapter 6, this volume).

All infants with intact skin are expected to be bathed by full immersion to the shoulder and neck level in suitably sized tubs filled with warm water. The infant may be placed in a deep warm water bath while loosely swaddled. Providing hands-on containment will further support an infant's relaxation and temperature stability. As soon and as frequently as possible, parents are the caregivers of choice to bathe their infant. Infants are expected to be weighed softly swaddled in a blanket or bunting, with gentle movement from bed to scale and back, unless the bed simultaneously provides a scale. All special examination and assessment procedures, including physical examinations, ultrasound examinations of the head, chest radiographs, EEGs, eye examinations, neurological examinations, and so on are performed collaboratively by the respective specialist and the infant's nurse, facilitated by the parent when possible, to support the infant's comfort and well-being in the course of required position changes, palpations, auscultations, and so forth. The infant's face is shielded whenever possible from intense illumination. At all times the size and quality of equipment, materials, and devices required are apportioned to the size and strength of the infant's limbs and skin to assure maximal comfort and physiologically appropriate alignment and movement of limbs and joints. Intravenous boards, whenever possible, support elbow flexion and finger grasp. Tape used is expected to be skin-friendly. When bilirubin blankets are not sufficient and bilirubin lights and eye patches are necessary, rest periods from eye covers should be provided with each caregiving interaction.

Enhancement of the Physical Environment in Support of Infants and Families

Lighting is adjusted to support each individual infant's and family's best sleep and awake organization and to deliver care without impinging on the development, comfort, and care of other infants. Individualized, controlled bedside lighting with dimmer capacity should be available. It is suggested that the general nursery lighting be indirect and readily adjusted in terms of brightness. Furthermore, nurseries should be quiet, soothing places. Suggestions for sound containment include creating a space within the NICU for admissions and special procedures; educating staff about preterm infant responses to various sound levels as part of the staff's training; moving daily rounds, discussions, and conversations away from infant and family bed spaces; dampening sounds from equipment, such as telephones, waste receptacles, monitor alarms, sinks, doors, and movable equipment; eliminating radios, overhead pagers, and all other unnecessary sound; transferring infants from warming tables to incubators with quiet motors as soon after admission as possible; covering incubators with thick blankets fitted with special sound-shielding material; choosing wall covering with sound-absorbent materials and structuring walls architecturally for maximal sound absorption; and carpeting all care areas.

Caregivers should avoid perfumes, colognes, and scented hair sprays, as infants are very sensitive to these odors. The odor of tobacco on caregivers' bodies and clothes as well as the odors of dry cleaning chemicals should also be avoided. Alcohol or sulfa-based chemicals should be used only while infants are removed from the care area. Cleaning fluid should dry and the vapors evaporate before bedding an infant back in the incubator. While parents are holding the infant skin-to-skin, a soft cloth placed across the infant and their own breasts or chests or a mother's breast pads will enhance and extend an infant's comfort in the recognition of the parent's odor when the infant is returned to the incubator, tucked in with the parents' cloth or pad.

The NICU environment is structured so that infants may be cared for in conjunction with their families. Specific aids such as sheepskin bedding, buntings, water mattresses, and pacifiers are used to lessen the impact of necessary medical procedures and equipment. Home-like, individualized spaces or family coves for infant and family within the NICU; secure, attractive cabinets to store belongings; communal space equipped with kitchen facilities; a library with written and audio-visual materials; washer and dryer facilities; rooms for sleeping; and bathroom and shower facilities for family members should be available. Twin and other multiple infants should be cared for in one family area and in one bed or incubator, if possible. Parents are encouraged to consider their infants' care spaces as their space. They are encouraged to arrange the space to their aesthetic liking. Bedside telephones for family members are of great importance for all families. The NICU should be structured for the 24-hour comfort not only of parents but also of the siblings and other family members. Family participation is facilitated by readily available, trained child-care provision for siblings. Siblings who pass a screen for exposure to Varicella and the presence of respiratory or other communicable illnesses present no increased risk to an infant. Since an infant's medical and nursing record (chart) are the parents' property, parents should be guided and encouraged to read the chart regularly and encouraged to enter their own observations and comments on a regular basis. This facilitates communication, builds mutual trust, and enhances the success of collaborative care.

Enhancement of Developmental Care Implementation

Implementation of developmental care in the NICU requires a multidisciplinary, collaborative approach. An analysis of the availability of resources and the unit's organizational functioning is an essential requirement prior to implementation of developmental care. Each infant has a primary team that includes the family and specific representatives from nursing, medicine, respiratory therapy, and social work, identified within the first 24 hours of its admission to the NICU. The primary team should work collaboratively to develop an individualized care plan, reviewed daily during rounds, which should include the parents, whenever possible. Regular team meetings should be scheduled. The family should be included to ensure their continued observations and input into their infant's plan of care.

Specially trained developmental professionals should be on staff full-time in each NICU as developmental clinicians. These professionals are expected to have knowledge of high-risk newborn and family development, as well as infant, parent, and professional mental health, and to support the primary teams in developmental care planning and implementation. They serve as resources and catalysts in developmental care collaboration. Institutions currently without developmental specialists should develop or acquire them and support the development of their role. The unitwide implementation of developmental care should be supported by a multidisciplinary developmental care committee. This committee focuses on coordinating unit-based developmental rounds, initiating a quality improvement project focusing on appropriate sound and light environments, organizing case presentations, developing a parent support group, and supporting developmental leadership in each of the NICU disciplines. A formal parent council with multicultural representation is suggested.

As the nursery moves to becoming a family-integrated living environment, the needs of nursery staff for private space should be considered very carefully. Resources and opportunities for personal and professional growth, such as regular meetings with a psychiatric clinical nurse specialist, psychiatrist, licensed clinical social worker, psychologist, or other mental health professional for the supportive discussion and reflection of family-staff and staff-staff issues, need to be provided. Ongoing collaboration with families to support their appreciation of and pride in their infants' strengths and individuality will prepare families for their infants' discharge from the NICU. Formal behavioral observation, using the NIDCAP® approach, in conjunction with formal assessment with the APIB, prior to an infant's discharge from the NICU or transfer to a community hospital, is recommended to support parents' and staff's understanding of its current behavioral functioning and to guide referrals to community services and early intervention programs.

SUMMARY

Reading the preterm infant and trusting its behavior as meaningful moves traditional newborn intensive care delivery into a collaborative, relationship-based neurodevelopmental framework. It leads to respect for infants and families as mutually attuned to and invested in one another. Infants and families are viewed as actively structuring their own development and engaging in continuous co-regulation with their physical and social environments. A developmental care framework highlights their mutually supportive striving to realize developmentally and individually specific expectations for the increasing differentiation and modulation of their own goals. These include autonomic, motor, and state system differentiation and modulation; feeding and elimination competence; and emotional, social, and cognitive efficacy and competence, all supporting ever greater differentiation of developing brain structures and species-specific functional competence.

Acknowledgments

This work was supported by grants GO-08720110 from the National Institute of Disability and Rehabilitation Research; HO-24590003 from the Office of Special Education Research, U.S. Department of Education; the Merck Family Fund; the Harris Foundation; and by grant P30 HD18655-12 from the National Institutes of Health, to J. J. Volpe. Appendix B is adapted from the *Manual for the Naturalistic Observation of Newborn Behavior*, by H. Als (Boston: Children's Hospital, 1984).

REFERENCES

Alberts, J. R., & Cramer, C. P. (1988). Ecology and experience: sources of means and meaning of developmental change. In E. M. Blass (Ed.), *Handbook of Behavioral Neurobiology: Developmental Psychobiology and Behavioral Ecology* (Vol. 9, pp. 1–40). New York: Plenum Press.

Allsopp, T. (1993). Life and death in the nervous system. *Trends Neurosci 16*, 1–4.

Als, H. (1975). The human newborn and his mother: an ethological study of their interaction [Ph.D. diss., University of Pennsylvania]. *Dissert Abs Int 36*, 5.

Als, H. (1977). The newborn communicates. *J Commun 27*, 66–73.

Als, H. (1978). Assessing an assessment: conceptual considerations, methodological issues, and a perspective on the future of the Neonatal Behavioral Assessment Scale. *MSCDA 43*, 14–28.

Als, H. (1979). Social interaction: dynamic matrix for developing behavioral organization. In I. C. Uzgiris (Ed.), *Social Interaction and Communication in Infancy: New Directions for Child Development* (pp. 21–41). San Francisco: Jossey-Bass.

Als, H. (1981). *Manual for the Naturalistic Observation of the Newborn (Preterm and Fullterm)*. Boston: Children's Hospital.

Als, H. (1982a). The behavior of the fetal newborn: theoretical considerations and practical suggestions for the use of the APIB. In C. E. Seashore, D. Lewis, & D. L. Saetveit (Eds.), *Issues in Neonatal Care. WESTAR* (pp. 19–60). Western States Technical Assistance Resource: Monmouth, Oregon.

Als, H. (1982b). Toward a synactive theory of development: Promise for the assessment of infant individuality. *Inf Mental Health J 3*, 229–243.

Als, H. (1982c). The unfolding of behavioral organization in the face of a biological violation. In E. Tronick (Ed.), *Human Communication and the Joint Regulation of Behavior* (pp. 125–160). Baltimore: University Park Press.

Als, H. (1983). Infant individuality: assessing patterns of very early development. In J. Call, E. Galenson, & R. L. Tyson (Eds.), *Frontiers of Infant Psychiatry* (pp. 363–378). New York: Basic Books.

Als, H. (1984). *Manual for the Naturalistic Observation of the Newborn (Preterm and Fullterm)* (rev.). Boston: Children's Hospital.

Als, H. (1986). A synactive model of neonatal behavioral organization: framework for the assessment and support of the neurobehavioral development of the premature infant and his parents in the environment of the neonatal intensive care unit. *Phys Occup Ther Pediatr 6*, 3–53.

Als, H. (1992). Individualized, family-focused developmental care for the very low birthweight preterm infant in the NICU. In S. L. Friedman & M. D. Sigman (Eds.), *Advances in Applied Developmental Psychology* (vol. 6, pp. 341–388). Norwood, NJ: Ablex.

Als, H. (1995). The preterm infant: a model for the study of fetal brain expectation. In J.-P. Lecanuet, W. P. Fifer, W. P. Smotherman, & N. A. Krasnegor (Eds.), *Fetal Development: A Psychobiological Perspective* (pp. 439–471). Hillsdale, NJ: Lawrence Erlbaum.

Als, H., & Berger, A. (1986). *Manual and Scoring System for the Assessment of Infants' Behavior: Kangaroo-Box Paradigm* (Unpublished manual). Boston: Children's Hospital.

Als, H., Duffy, F. H., & McAnulty, G. B. (In preparation). Longterm effects of very early individualized developmental care in the NICU to 3 and 7 years post term.

Als, H., Duffy, F. H., & McAnulty, G. B. (In press). Neurobehavioral competence in healthy preterm and fullterm infants: Newborn period to 9 months. *Dev Psychol*.

Als, H., Duffy, F. H., McAnulty, G., & Badian, N. (1989). Continuity of neurobehavioral functioning in preterm and fullterm newborns. In M. H. Bornstein & N. A. Krasnegor (Eds.), *Stability and Continuity in Mental Development* (pp. 3–28). Hillsdale, NJ: Lawrence Erlbaum.

Als, H., & Gilkerson, L. (1989–1994). National collaborative research institute for early childhood intervention: family-focused developmental care and intervention for the very low birthweight preterm infant at high risk for severe medical complication and developmental disabilities (Unpublished manuscript, Children's Hospital). Boston: U.S. Department of Education, OSERS, EEPCD.

Als, H., Lawhon, G., Brown, E., Gibes, R., Duffy, F. H., McAnulty, G. B., & Blickman, J. G. (1986). Individualized behavioral and environmental care for the very low birth weight preterm infant at high risk for bronchopulmonary dysplasia: Neonatal Intensive Care Unit and developmental outcome. *Pediatrics 78*, 1123–1132.

Als, H., Lawhon, G., Duffy, F. H., McAnulty, G. B., Gibes-Grossman, R., & Blickman, J. G. (1994). Individualized developmental care for the very low birthweight preterm infant: medical and neurofunctional effects. *JAMA 272*, 853–858.

Als, H., Lawhon, G., Melzar, A., Duffy, F. H., McAnulty, G. B., & Blickman, J. G. (In preparation). Individualized behavioral and developmental care for the VLBW preterm infant at high risk for bronchopulmonary dysplasia and intraventricular hemorrhage: study III: a clinical model.

Als, H., Lester, B. M., & Brazelton, T. B. (1979). Dynamics of the behavioral organization of the premature infant: a theoretical perspective. In T. M. Field, A. M. Sostek, S. Goldberg, & H. H. Shuman (Eds.), *Infants Born at Risk* (pp. 173–193). New York: Spectrum.

Als, H., Lester, B. M., Tronick, E. Z., & Brazelton, T. B. (1982a). Manual for the assessment of preterm infants' behavior (APIB). In H. E. Fitzgerald, B. M. Lester, & M. W. Yogman (Eds.), *Theory and Research in Behavioral Pediatrics* (vol. 1, pp. 65–132). New York: Plenum Press.

Als, H., Lester, B. M., Tronick, E. Z., & Brazelton, T. B. (1982b). Towards a research instrument for the assessment of preterm infants' behavior. In H. E. Fitzgerald, B. M. Lester, & M. W. Yogman (Eds.), *Theory and Research in Behavioral Pediatrics* (vol. 1, pp. 35–63). New York: Plenum Press.

Anderson, G. C., Burroughs, A. K., & Measel, C. P. (1983). Non-nutritive sucking opportunities: a safe and effective treatment for preterm neonates. In T. Field & A. Sostek (Eds.), *Infants Born at Risk* (pp. 129–147). New York: Grune and Stratton.

Andrew, R. J. (1963a). Evolution of facial expression. *Science 142*, 1034–1041.

Andrew, R. J. (1963b). The origin and evolution of the cells and facial expressions of primates. *Behavior 20*, 1–109.

Avery, M. E., Tooley, W. H., Keller, J. B., Hurd, S. S., Bryan, H., Cotton, R. B., Epstein, M. F., Fitzhardinge, P. M., Hansen, C. B., Hansen, T. N., Hodson, A., James, L. S., Kitterman, J. A., Nielsen, H. C., Poirier, T. A., Truog, W. E., & Wiung, J. T. (1987). Is chronic lung disease in low birth weight infants preventable: a survey of eight centers. *Pediatrics 79*, 26–30.

Babson, S. G. (1970). Growth of low birthweight infants. *J Pediatr 77*, 11–18.

Becker, P. T., Grunwald, P. C., Moorman, J., & Stuhr, S. (1991). Outcomes of developmentally supportive nursing care for very low birthweight infants. *Nurs Res 40*, 150–155.

Becker, P. T., Grunwald, P. C., Moorman, J., & Stuhr, S. (1993). Effects of developmental care on behavioral organization in very-low-birth-weight infants. *Nurs Res 42*, 214–220.

Birnholz, J. C. (1988). On observing the human fetus. In W. P. Smotherman & S. R. Robinson (Eds.), *Behavior of the Fetus* (pp. 47–62). Caldwell, NJ: Telford Press.

Blurton Jones, N. (1972). Characteristics of ethological studies of human behavior. In N. Blurton Jones (Ed.), *Ethological Studies of Child Behavior* (pp. 3–37). Cambridge: Cambridge University Press.

Blurton Jones, N. (1974). Ethology and early socialization. In M. P. M. Richards (Ed.), *The Integration of a Child into a Social World* (pp. 263–295). Cambridge: Cambridge University.

Blurton Jones, N. (1976). Growing points in human ethology: another link between ethology and the social sciences. In P. P. G. Bateson & R. A. Hinde (Eds.), *Growing Points in Ethology* (pp. 427–451). Cambridge: Cambridge University Press.

Bolwig, N. (1959a). Observations and thoughts on the evolution of facial mimic. *Koedoe 2*, 60–69.

Bolwig, N. (1959b). A study of the behavior of the chacma baboon, *Papio ursinus. 14*, 136–163.

Bolwig, N. (1964). Facial expression in primates with remarks on a parallel development in certain carnivores. *Behavior 23*, 167–193.

Bourgeois, J. P., Jastreboff, P. J., & Rakic, P. (1989). Synaptogenesis in visual cortex of normal and preterm monkeys: evidence for intrinsic regulation of synaptic overproduction. *Proc Natl Acad Sci USA 86*, 4297–4301.

Brazelton, T. B. (1973). *Neonatal Behavioral Assessment Scale*. London: Heinemann.

Brazelton, T. B. (1984). *Neonatal Behavioral Assessment Scale*. (2nd ed.). Philadelphia: Spastics International Medical Publications, Lippincott.

Brazelton, T. B., & Als, H. (1979). Four early stages in the development of mother-infant interaction. *Psychoanal Study Child 34*, 349–369.

Buehler, D. M., Als, H., Duffy, F. H., McAnulty, G. B., & Liederman, J. (1995). Effectiveness of individualized developmental care for low-risk preterm infants: behavioral and electrophysiological evidence. *Pediatrics 96*, 923–932.

Buettner-Janusch, J. (1966). *Origins of Man*. New York: John Wiley.

Burroughs, A. K., Asonye, U. O., Anderson-Shanklin, G. C., & Vidyasagar, D. (1978). The effect of non-nutritive sucking on transcutaneous oxygen tension in non-crying preterm neonates. *Res Nurs Health 1*, 69–75.

Catsicas, S., Thanos, S., & Clarke, P. G. (1987). Major role for neuronal death during brain development: refinement of topographical connections. *Proc Natl Acad Sci USA 84*, 8165–8168.

Chaudhari, S., Kulkarni, S., Pajnigar, F., Pandit, A. N., & Deshmukh, S. (1991). A longitudinal follow up of development of preterm infants. *Ind Pediatr 28*, 873–880.

Cornell, E. H., & Gottfried, A. W. (1976). Intervention with premature human infants. *Child Dev 47*, 32–39.

Cowan, F., & Thoresen, M. (1985). Changes in superior sagittal sinus blood velocities due to postural alterations and pressure on the head of the newborn infant. *Pediatrics 75(6)*, 1038–1047.

Cowan, W. M. (1979). The development of the brain. In *The Brain. A Scientific American Book* (pp. 56–67). San Francisco: W. H. Freeman.

Cupoli, J. M., Gagan, R. J., Watkins, A. H., & Bell, S. F. (1986). The shapes of grief. *J Perinatol* 6(2), 123–126.

Danford, D. A., Miske, S., Headley, J., & Nelson, R. M. (1983). Effects of routine care procedures on transcutaneous oxygen in neonates: a quantitative approach. *Arch Dis Child 58*, 20–23.

De Carlos, J. A., & O'Leary, D. M. (1992). Growth and targeting of subplate axons and establishment of major cortical pathways. *J Neurosci 12*, 1194–1211.

de Vries, J. I. P., Visser, G. H. A., & Prechtl, H. F. R. (1982). The emergence of fetal behavior. I. Qualitative Aspects. *Early Hum Dev 7*, 301–322.

de Vries, J. I. P., Visser, G. H. A., & Prechtl, H. F. R. (1988). The emergence of fetal behavior. III. Individual differences and consistencies. *Early Hum Dev 16*, 85–104.

de Vries, L. S., Dubowitz, L. M. S., Dubowitz, V., Kaiser, A., Lary, S., Silverman, M., Whitelaw, A., & Wigglesworth, J. S. (1985). Predictive value of cranial ultrasound in the newborn baby: a reappraisal. *Lancet 2*, 137–140.

Denckla, M. B. (1993). The child with developmental disabilities grown up: adult residua of childhood disorders. *Neurol Clin 11*, 105–125.

Denny-Brown, D. (1962). *The Basal Ganglia and Their Relation to Disorders of Movement*. Oxford: Oxford University Press.

Denny-Brown, D. (1966). *The Cerebral Control of Movement*. Springfield, IL: Charles C Thomas.

Dooling, E. C., Chi, J. G., & Gilles, F. H. (1983). Telencephalic development: changing gyral patterns. In F. H. Gilles, A. Leviton, & E. C. Dooling (Eds.), *The Developing Human Brain* (pp. 94–104). Boston: John Wright.

Driscoll, M., & Chalfie, M. (1992). Developmental and abnormal cell death in *C. elegans. Trends Neurosci 15*, 15–19.

Duffy, F. H., Als, H., & McAnulty, G. B. (1990). Behavioral and electrophysiological evidence for gestational age effects in healthy preterm and fullterm infants studied 2 weeks after expected due date. *Child Dev 61*, 1271–1286.

Duffy, F. H., & Burchfiel, J. L. (1971). Somato-sensory systems: organizational hierarchy from single units in monkey area 5. *Science 172*, 273–275.

Duffy, F. H., & Burchfiel, J. L., & Lombroso, C. T. (1979). Brain electrical activity mapping (BEAM): a method for extending the clinical utility of EEG and evoked potential data. *Ann Neurol 5*, 309–321.

Duffy, F. H., Burchfiel, J. L., & Snodgrass, S. R. (1978). The pharmacology of amblyopia. *Arch Ophthalmol 85*, 489–495.

Duffy, F. H., Mower, G. D., Jensen, F., & Als, H. (1984). Neural plasticity: a new frontier for infant development. In H. E. Fitzgerald, B. M. Lester, & M. W. Yogman (Eds.), *Theory and Research in Behavioral Pediatrics* (vol. 2, pp. 67–96). New York: Plenum Press.

Easter, S. S., Purves, D., Rakic, P., & Spitzer, N. C. (1985). The changing view of neural specificity. *Science 230*, 507–511.

Erikson, E. H. (1962). Reality and actualization. *J Am Psychoanal Assoc 10*, 451–475.

Ferrer, I., Soriano, E., & Delrio, J. A. (1992). Cell death and removal in the cerebral cortex during development. *Prog Neurobiol 39*, 1–43.

Field, T. M., Ignatoff, E., Stringer, S., Brennan, J., Greenberg, R., Widmayer, S., & Anderson, G. C. (1982). Non-nutritive sucking during tube feedings: effects on preterm neonates in an intensive care unit. *Pediatrics 70* 381–384.

Finlay, B. L., & Miller, B. (1993). Regressive events in early cortical maturation: their significance for theoutcome of early brain damage. In A. M. Galaburda (Ed.), *Dyslexia and Development*, (pp. 1–21). Cambridge, MA: Harvard University Press.

Fischer, K. W., & Rose, S. P. (1994). Dynamic development of coordination of components in brain and behavior: a framework for theory and research. In G. Dawson & K. W. Fischer (Eds.), *Human Behavior and the Developing Brain* (pp. 3–66). New York: Guilford Press.

Fleisher, B. F., VandenBerg, K. A., Constantinou, J., Heller, C., Benitz, W. E., Johnson, A., Rosenthal, A., & Stevenson, D. K. (1995). Individualized developmental care for very-low-birth-weight premature infants. *Clin Pediatr, 34*, 523–529.

Freud, W. E. (1991). Das "Whose Baby" Syndrom. Ein Beitrag zum psychodynamischen Verständnis der Perinatologie. In M. Stauger, F. Conrad, & G. Haselbacher (Eds.), *Psychosomatische Gynäkologie und Geburtshilfe*, (pp. 123–137). Berlin: Springer-Verlag.

Galaburda, A. M., & Kemper, T. L. (1979). Cytoarchitectonic abnormalities in developmental dyslexia: a case study. *Ann Neurol, 6*, 94–100.

Gesell, A., & Armatruda, C. (1945). *The Embryology of Behavior*. Westport, CT: Connecticut Greenwood Press.

Ghosh, A., & Shatz, C. J. (1993). A role for subplate neurons in the patterning of connections from thalamus to neocortex. *Development, 117*, 1031–1047.

Gilles, F. H. (1983). Changes in growth and vulnerability at the end of the second trimester. In A. Gilles, A. Leviton, & E. C. Dooling (Eds.), *The Developing Human Brain* (pp. 316–320). Boston: John Wright.

Gilles, F. H., Leviton, A., & Dooling, E. C. (1983a). *The Developing Human Brain*. Boston: John Wright.

Gilles, F. H., Shankle, W., Dooling, E. C. (1983b). Myelinated tracts: growth patterns. In F. H. Gilles, A. Leviton, & E. C. Dooling (Eds.), *The Developing Human Brain* (pp. 117–184). Boston: John Wright.

Gong, A. K., Van Heuven, W. A. J., Berlanga, M., & Escobedo, M. B. (1989). Severe retinopathy in convalescent preterm infants with mild or regressing retinopathy of prematurity. *Pediatrics, 83*, 422–425.

Gorski, P. A., Hole, W. T., Leonard, C. H., & Martin, J. A. (1983). Direct computer recording of premature infants and nursery care: distress following two interventions. *Pediatrics, 72*, 198–202.

Gottfried, A. W., & Gaiter, J. L. (1985). *Infant Stress Under Intensive Care*. Baltimore: University Park Press.

Grossman, K. (1978). Die Wirkung des Augenoffnens von Neugeborenen auf das Verhalten ihrer Mutter. *Geburtshilfe und Frauenheilkunde, 38*, 629–635.

Grunwald, P. C., & Becker, P. T. (1990). Developmental enhancement: implementing a program for the NICU. *Neonatal Network, 9* (6), 29–45.

Guyer, B., Strobino, D. M., Ventura, S. J., MacDorman, M., & Martin, J. A. (1996). Annual summary of vital statistics—1995. *Pediatrics, 98* (6), 1007–1019.

Hack, M., Taylor, G., Klein, N., Eiben, R., Schatschneider, C., & Mercuri-Minich, N. (1994). School-age outcomes in children with birth weights under 750 g. *N Engl J Med, 331*, 753–759.

Hansen, N., & Okken, A. (1979). Continuous TcPO2 monitoring in healthy and sick newborn infants during and after feeding. *Birth Defects, 4*, 503–508.

Hassenstein, B. (1973). *Verhaltungsbiologie des Kindes*. Munich: Piper Verlag.

Hepper, P., & Shahidullah, S. (1992). Abnormal fetal behavior in Down's Syndrome fetuses. *Q J Clin Psych, 44*, 305–317.

Heuman, D., & Leuba, G. (1983). Neuronal death in the development and aging of the cerebral cortex of the mouse. *Neuropathol Appl Neurobiol, 9*, 297–311.

Hofer, M. A. (1987). Early social relationships: a psychobiologist's view. *Child Dev, 58*, 633–647.

Holmes, M., Sheldon, R., & Als, H. (1995). *Developmentally supportive and family centered care: Newborn Intensive Care Unit participation standards* (Unpublished manuscript). Oklahoma City: University of Oklahoma Health Sciences Center.

Huber, E. (1931). *Evolution of Facial Musculature and Facial Expression.* Baltimore: Johns Hopkins Press.

Humphrey, T. (1964). Some correlations between the appearance of human fetal reflexes and the development of the nervous system. *Prog Brain Res, 4*, 93–135.

Hunt, J. V., Cooper, B. A. B., & Tooley, W. H. (1988). Very low birth weight infants at 8 and 11 years of age: role of neonatal illness and family status. *Pediatrics, 82*, 596–603.

Hunt, J. V., Tooley, W. H., & Cooper, B. A. B. (1992). Further investigations of intellectual status at age 8 years: I. Long-term consequences into adulthood. II. Neonatal predictors. In S. L. Friedman & M. D. Sigman (Eds.), *Advances in Applied Developmental Psychology, Volume 6. The Psychological Developmental of Low Birthweight Children* (pp. 315–337). Norwood, NJ: Ablex.

Hunt, J. V., Tooley, W. H., & Harvin, D. (1982). Learning disabilities in children with birthweights < 1,500 grams. *Semin Perinatol, 6*, 280–287.

Huttenlocher, P. R. (1984). Synapse elimination and plasticity in developing human cerebral cortex. *Am J Ment Defic, 88*, 488–496.

Ianniruberto, A., & Tajani, E. (1981). Ultrasonographic study of fetal movements. *Semin Perinatol, 5*, 175–181.

Klaus, M. H. (1982). Application of recent findings to clinical care. In M. H. Klaus & M. O. Robertson (Eds.), *Birth, Interaction, and Attachment* (6th ed., pp. 129–134): Johnson and Johnson Pediatric Roundtable.

Klaus, M., & Kennel, J. H. (1982). *Parent-Infant Bonding.* St. Louis: Mosby.

Kliegman, R. M., & Walsh, M. C. (1987). Neonatal necrotizing enterocolitis: pathogenesis, classification, and spectrum of illness. *Curr Probl Pediatr, 17*, 213–288.

Largo, R. M., Molinari, L., Kundu, S., Lipp, A., & Duc, G. (1990). Intellectual outcome, speech and school performance in high risk preterm children with birth weight appropriate for gestational age. *Eur J Pediatr, 149*, 845–850.

Larroche, J.-C. (1981). The marginal zone in the neocortex of a 7-week-old human embryo. *Anat Embryo, 162*, 301–312.

Lawhon, G. (1986). Management of stress in premature infants. In D. J. Angelini, C. M. Whelan Knapp, & R. M. Gibes (Eds.), *Perinatal Neonatal Nursing: A Clinical Handbook*, (pp. 319–328). Boston: Blackwell Scientific Publications.

Lawhon, G., & Melzar, A. (1991). Developmentally supportive interventions. In J. P. Cloherty & A. R. Stark (Eds.), *Manual of Neonatal Care* (3rd ed., pp. 581–584). Boston: Little, Brown.

Lettvin, J. Y., Maturana, H., McCulloch, W., & Pitts, W. (1959). What the frog's eye tells the frog's brain. *Proc I Radio Engineers, 47*, 1940–1951.

Leviton, A., & Gilles, F. H. (1983). The epidemiology of delayed myelination. In F. H. Gilles, A. Leviton, & E. C. Dooling (Eds.), *The Developing Human Brain* (pp. 185–203). Boston: John Wright.

Lewis, M. E., Mishkin, M., Bragin, E., Brown, R. M., Pert, C. B., & Pert, A. (1981). Opiate receptor gradients in monkey cerebral cortex: correspondence with sensory processing hierarchies. *Science, 211*, 1166–1169.

Liaw, F. R., & Brooks-Gunn, J. (1993). Patterns of low-weight children's cognitive development. *Dev. Psychol, 29*, 1024–1035.

Linn, P. L., Horowitz, F. D., Buddin, B. J., Leake, J. C., & Fox, H. A. (1985). Stimulation in the NICU: is more necessarily better? *Clin Perinatol, 12*, 407–422.

Littman, B., & Parmelee, A. H. (1974). *Manual for Obstetric Complications* (Unpublished manual). Los Angeles: Infant Studies Project, Department of Pediatrics, School of Medicine, University of California, Los Angeles.

Long, J. G., Lucey, J. F., & Philip, A. G. S. (1980). Noise and hypoxemia in the intensive care nursery. *Pediatrics, 65*, 143–145.

Long, J. G., Philip, A. G. S., & Lucey, J. F. (1980). Excessive handling as a cause of hypoxemia. *Pediatrics, 65(2)*, 203–207.

Marin-Padilla, M. (1983). Structural organization of the human cerebral cortex prior to the appearance of the cortical plate. *Anat Embryo, 168*, 21–40.

Marin-Padilla, M. (1993). Pathogenesis of late-acquired leptomeningeal heterotopias and secondary cortical alterations: a golgi study. In A. M. Galaburda (Ed.), *Dyslexia and Development* (pp. 64–89). Cambridge, MA: Harvard University Press.

Martin, R. J., Herrell, N., Rubin, D., & Fanaroff, A. (1979). Effect of supine and prone positions on arterial oxygen tension in the preterm infant. *Pediatrics, 63*, 528–531.

Martin, R. J., Okken, A., & Rubin, D. (1979). Arterial oxygen tension during active and quiet sleep in the normal neonate. *J Pediatr, 94*, 271–274.

Maus, A., & Endresen, J. (1979). Misuse of computer-generated results. *Med Biol Eng Comput, 17*, 126–129.

McConnell, S. K., Ghosh, A., & Shatz, C. J. (1989). Subplate neurons pioneer the first axon pathway from the cerebral cortex. *Science, 245*, 978–982.

McCormick, M. C. (1992). Advances in neonatal intensive care technology and their possible impact on the development of low birthweight infants. In S. L. Friedman & M. D. Sigman (Eds.), *The Psychological Development of Low-Birthweight Children. Advances in Applied Developmental Psychology* (pp. 37–60). Norwood, NJ: Ablex.

McLennan, J. E., Gilles, F. H., & Neff, R. (1983). A model of growth of the human fetal brain. In F. H. Gilles, A. Leviton, & D. C. Dooling (Eds.), *The Developing Human Brain* (pp. 43–59). Boston: John Wright.

Minde, K., Morton, P., Manning, D., & Hines, B. (1980). Some determinants of mother-infant interaction in the premature nursery. *J Am Ac Child Psych, 19*, 1–21.

Minde, K., Trehub, S., Carter, C., Boukydis, C., Celhoffer, L., & Morton, P. (1978). Mother-child relationships in the premature nursery: an observation study. *Pediatrics, 61*, 373–379.

Minde, K., Whitelaw, A., Brown, J., & Fitzhardinge, P. (1983). Effect of neonatal complications in premature infants on early parent-child interactions. *Dev Med Child Neurol, 25*, 763–777.

Mower, G. D., Burchfiel, J. L., & Duffy, F. H. (1982). Animal models of strabismic amblyopia: physiological studies of visual cortex and the lateral geniculate nucleus. *Dev Brain Res 5*, 311–327.

Murdoch, D. R., & Darlow, B. A. (1984). Handling during neonatal intensive care. *Arch Dis Childhood, 29*, 957–961.

Nilsson, L. (1973). *Behold Man*. Boston: Little, Brown.

Norris, S., Campbell, L., & Brenkert, S. (1982). Nursing procedures and alterations in transcutaneous oxygen tension in premature infants. *Nurs Res, 31*, 330–336.

O'Brodovich, H., & Mellins, R. (1985). Bronchopulmonary dysplasia. Unresolved neonatal acute lung injury. *Am Rev Respir Dis, 132*, 694–709.

Oberklaid, F., Sewall, J., Sanson, A., & Prior, M. (1991). Temperament and behavior of preterm infants: a six-year follow-up. *Pediatrics, 87*, 854–861.

Oppenheim, R. W. (1991). Cell death during development of the nervous system. *Annu Rev Neurosci, 14*, 453–501.

Oppenheim, R. W., Schwartz, L. M., & Shatz, C. J. (1992). Neuronal death, a tradition of dying. *J Neurobiol, 23*, 1111–1115.

Prechtl, H. F. R. (1977). *The Neurological Examination of the Full Term Infant: A Manual for Clinical use*. (2nd ed.). Philadelphia: Lippincott.

Purves, D., & Lichtman, J. W. (1980). Elimination of synapses in the developing nervous system. *Science, 210*, 153–157.

Rakic, P. (1988). Specification of cerebral cortical areas. *Science, 241*, 170–176.

Rakic, P. (1990). Principles of neural cell migration. *Experientia, 46*, 882–891.

Rakic, P. (1991). Experimental manipulation of cerebral cortical areas in primates. *Philos Trans Royal Soc London, 331*, 291–294.

Rakic, P., Suñer, I., & Williams, R. W. (1991). A novel cytoarchitectonic area induced experimentally within the primate visual cortex. *Proc NA Sci, 88*, 2083–2087.

Reppert, S. M., & Rivkees, S. A. (1989). Development of human circadian rhythms: implications for health and disease. In S. M. Reppert (Ed.), *Development of Circadian Rhythmicity and Photoperiodism in Mammals* (Research in Perinatal Medicine, Vol. 9, pp. 245–259). Ithaca, NY: Perinatology Press.

Robson, K. (1967). The role of eye-to-eye contact in maternal-infant attachment. *J Child Psych & Psychiatry, 8*, 13–25.

Rosen, G. D., Sherman, G. F., & Galaburda, A. M. (1993). Dyslexia and brain pathology: experimental animal models. In A. M. Galaburda (Ed.), *Dyslexia and Development* (pp. 89–111). Cambridge, MA: Harvard University Press.

Rosenblatt, J. S. (1976). Stages in the early behavioral development of altricial young of selected species of non-primate mammals. In P. P. G. Bateson & R. A. Hinde (Eds.), *Growing Points in Ethology*. Cambridge University Press.

Sander, L. W. (1962). Issues in early mother-child interaction *J Am Acad C Psych, 1*, 141–166.

Sander, L. W. (1964). Adaptive relationships in early mother-child interaction. *J Am Acad Child Psychiatry, 3*, 231–264.

Sander, L. W. (1970). Regulation and organization in the early infant-caretaker system. In R. Robinson (Ed.), *Brain and Early Behavior* (pp. 311–333). London: Academic Press.

Sander, L. W. (1975). Infant and caretaking environment: investigation and conceptualization of adaptive behavior in a system of increasing complexity. In E. J. Anthony (Ed.), *Explorations in child psychiatry*. New York: Plenum Press.

Sander, L. W. (1976). Primary prevention and some aspects of temporal organization in early infant-caretaker interaction. In E. Rexford, L. W. Sander, & T. Shapiro (Eds.), *Infant Psychiatry: A New Synthesis* (pp. 187–204). New Haven, CT: Yale.

Sander, L. W. (1980). Investigation of the infant and its environment as a biological system. In S. I. Greenberg & G. H. Pollock (Eds.), *The Course of Life: Psyoanalytic Contribution Toward Understanding Personality Development* (pp. 177–201). Washington, DC: National Institute of Mental Health.

Sander, L. W., Stechler, G., Burns, P., & Lee, A. (1979). Change in infant and caregiver variables over the first two months of life: integration of action in early development. In E. B. Thomas (Ed.), *Origins of the Infant's Social Responsiveness*. Hillsdale, NJ: Lawrence Erlbaum.

Schade, J. P., & van Groenigen, D. B. (1961). Structural organization of the human cerebral cortex. I. Maturation of the middle frontal gyrus. *Act Anat, 41*, 47–111.

Schneirla, T. C. (1959). An evolutionary and developmental theory of biphasic processes underlying approach and withdrawal. In M. R. Jones (Ed.), *Nebraska Symposium on Motivation* (pp. 1 42). Lincoln: University of Nebraska Press.

Schneirla, T. C. (1965). Aspects of stimulation and organization in approach and withdrawal processes underlying vertebrate development. *Adv Study of Behav, 1*, 1–74.

Schneirla, T. C., & Rosenblatt, J. S. (1961). Behavioral organization and genesis of the social bond in insects and mammals. *Am J Orthopsychiat, 31*, 223–253.

Schneirla, T. C., & Rosenblatt, J. S. (1963). "Critical periods" in the development of behavior. *Science, 139*, 1110–1115.

Sostek, A. M. (1992). Prematurity as well as intraventricular hemorrhage influence developmental outcome at 5 years. In S. L. Friedman & M. D. Sigman (Eds.), *Advances in Applied developmental Psychology, Volume 6. The Psychological Development of Low Birthweight Children* (pp. 259–274). Norwood, NJ: Ablex.

Spinelli, D. N., Jensen, F. E., & DePrisco, G. V. (1980). Early experience effect on dendritic branchings in normally reared kittens. *Exper Neurol, 68*, 1–11.

Springate, J. E. (1981). The neuroanatomic basis of early motor development: a review. *Dev Behav Ped, 2*, 146–150.

Tajani, E., & Ianniruberto, A. (1990). The uncovering of fetal "competence." In M. Papini, A. Pasquinelli, & E. A. Gidoni (Eds.), *Development, Handicap, Rehabilitation: Practice and Theory*. Amsterdam: Elsevier.

Turkewitz, G., & Kenney, P. A. (1985). The role of developmental limitations of sensory input on sensory/perceptual organization. *J Dev Behav Ped, 6*, 302–306.

Valman, H. B., & Pearson, J. P. (1980). What the fetus feels. *Brit Med J, 280*, 233–234.

VandenBerg, K. A. (1990a). Behaviorally supportive care for the extremely premature infant. In L. P. Gunderson & C. Kenner (Eds.), *Care of the 24–25 Week Gestational Age Infant (Small Baby Protocol)* (pp. 129–157). Petaluma, CA-Neonatal Network.

VandenBerg, K. A. (1990b). Nippling management of the sick neonate in the NICU: the disorganized feeder. *Neonatal Network, 9(1)*, 9–16.

VandenBerg, K. A., & Franck, L. S. (1990). Behavioral issues for infants with BPD. In C. Lund (Ed.), *BPD: Strategies for Total Patient Care* (pp. 113–152). Petaluma, CA: Neonatal Network.

Vento, T., & Feinberg, E. (In press). Developmentally supportive care. In J. Cloherty & A. Stark (Eds.), *Developmentally Supportive Care (4th Edition)* ed., Boston: Little, Brown.

Volpe, J. J. (1989a). Intraventricular hemorrhage in the premature infant—current concepts. Part I. *Ann Neurol, 25(1)*, 3–11.

Volpe, J. J. (1989b). Intraventricular hemorrhage in the premature infant—current concepts. Part II. *Ann Neurol, 25(2)*, 109–116.

Volpe, J. J. (1995). *Neurology of the Newborn* (3rd ed.). Philadelphia: W. B. Saunders.

Waber, D. P., McCormick, M. C., & Workman-Daniels, K. (1992). *Neurobehavioral outcomes in very low birthweight, low birthweight, and normal birthweight children with and without medical complications*. Abstract presented at the International Neuropsychological Society 21st Annual Meeting, Galveston, Texas.

Walsh, C., & Cepko, C. L. (1992). Widespread dispersion of neuronal clones across functional regions of the cerebral cortex. *Science, 255*, 434–440.

Willis, W. D., & Grossman, R. G. (1981). *Medical Neurobiology*. St. Louis: C. V. Mosby.

Wolke, D. (1987). Environmental and developmental neonatology. *J Repr Inf Psychol, 5*, 17–42.

Yakovlev, P. I., & Lecours, A. R. (1967). The myelogenic cycles of regional maturation of the brain. In A. Minkowsky (Ed.), *Regional Development of the Brain in Early Life* (pp. 3–70). Oxford: Blackwell.

APPENDIX A: CASE REPORT

Behavioral Observation

Introduction

Robert was observed at the Newborn Intensive Care Unit at St. L. Hospital in the context of a teaching session. The observation (Fig. A1) took place March 1, 1995, 8:12 AM–8:52 AM. Robert's nurse was observed in interaction with Robert. Four observers participated in the teaching session (Fig. A2).

Observation

1. Nursery Environment

   Robert's incubator was in Room 3, a large rectangular care room with big windows along one of the long and one of the short walls of the room. There were eleven beds lined up along the long walls of the room; ten were occupied. Several of the infants were cared for in incubators, two were in open cribs, and the infant immediately adjacent to Robert was on an open warming table; his breathing was supported with a special high frequency ventilator, which made continuous loud sounds. Robert's incubator was directly under one of the large windows and immediately across the open room door leading to the hallway. Bright sunlight streamed through the windows. Staff members quietly walked back and forth, shielding their eyes from the sun with their hands. A few window blinds were partially pulled. All overhead ceiling lights were on. At times up to 10 staff members and several parents were in the room, engaged in various activities; refuse bins were being emptied; alarms sounded; a telephone rang repeatedly; voice levels rose and fell in cycles. At the foot of each bed was a large cabinet; this narrowed the main passage between the incubators and cribs so that only one person at a time could pass along the center aisle of the room. Some of the incubators were covered with soft quilts, others with blankets. Chairs were available at some of the bedsides. Overall, the room was full of activity and space appeared tight, although relatively well organized.

2. Robert's Bedspace and Bedding

   Robert was bedded on his tummy on a sheepskin-covered mattress supported by a blanket roll for his feet and along his sides and head. He faced to his left, his eyes shielded with a mask to protect him from the special bright lights (bilirubin lights) above him used to treat his jaundice. His buttocks were tucked up, yet his knees were out beside his hips and his

NATURALISTIC OBSERVATION OF NEWBORN BEHAVIOR
(NIDCAP)

Name of Infant _ROBERT A._

Sex _MALE_

Hospital & Record # _ST. L. H._

MATERNAL HISTORY

Prepregnancy Health _HYPERTENSION; VAGINAL_

Pregnancy _BLEEDING; THREAT OF ABRUPTED PLACENTA;_

Labor & Delivery _3 DAYS HOSPITALIZATION, TERBUTALINE_

Medications _DEXAMETHASONE_

Other (G/P) _G3 - P3_

INFANT HISTORY

DOB _FEB 26, 1995_ EDC _MAY 5, 1995_

Post LMP Age at Birth _29.5_ weeks_____ days

Mode of Delivery _VAGINAL_

Apgars _5_ 1 min _7_ 5 min _-_ 10 min

Birthweight _1340_ g _50_ %

Length at Birth _38_ cm _50_ %

Head Circ at Birth _28_ cm _75_ %

PI _2.44_ ; _60_ %

AGA ☒ SGA ☐ LGA ☐

Other _____

Respiratory Function:

Respirator ☐ _____ No. of Days

CPAP ☒ _14 HRS._ No. of Days

Oxyhood ☒ _8 HRS._ No. of Days

Nas. Cannula ☐ _____ No. of Days

Hi Insp O$_2$ _____

No Aid ☒ _SINCE 22 HRS IN ROOM AIR_

Other _____

Medications:

Sedatives _1 DOSE OF VERCET_

Bronchodilators _____

Diuretics _____

Anticonvulsants _____

Steroids _____

Antibiotics _1 DOSE OF VANCOMYCIN_

Other _CAFFEINE 1 × DAY_

Mode of Feeding: _FOR 12 hrs, then NPO_

IV ☒ Gavage: Nasal ☒ Oral ☐

Bottle ☐ Breast ☐ _HYPERAL & LIPIDS_

Type: Breast Milk ☐ Formula ☐ _____ Cal

Caregiving Interval _Q3 → Q4_ ⎱

Feeding Interval _____ ⎰

Other _____

Complications:

Asphyxia ☐   RDS ☐   BPD ☐

Sepsis ☐   A&B ☐   NEC ☐

IVH ☐   Grade R _____ /L _____

ROP ☐   Stage R _____ /L _____

PDA ☒   Med/Surgery _INDOCIN × 2_

Bili (HI) _✓_ Lights (Type) _✓_

Ostomy _____

Surgery _____

Date _1 MARCH 1995_

Name of Observer _K.S., M.R, D.S., H.A._

Parents' Names, Address, and Telephone No. _____

JUDY A.

Mother's Age _31_ Father's Age _?_

Family Situation _NOT YET COMPLETELY CLARIFIED_

Other Children _2_ Ages _9 yrs, 7 yrs._

CURRENT STATUS

Age Post LMP _30_ wks _-_ days

Age Post Birth _-_ wks _4_ days

Weight _?_ g ____ % Height _?_ cm ____ %

Head Circ _?_ cm ____ % PI _?_ ; ____ %

Respiratory Function:

Respirator ☐ _-_ FIO$_2$

Oxyhood ☐ _-_ FIO$_2$

CPAP ☐ _-_

Nasal Cannula _-_ ☐ cc____ FIO$_2$

Insp O$_2$ Req'd (prec 24hrs) _ROOM AIR_

Mean FIO$_2$ _-_ Mean PCO$_2$ _-_

Mean MAP _-_ Heartrate (Range) _?_

O$_2$ Sats (Range) _?_ Resp. Rate (Range) _?_

Medications: _CAFFEINE_

_____

_____

Mode of Feeding:

IV ☐ Gavage: Nasal ☐ Oral ☐

Bottle ☐ Breast ☐

Type: Breast Milk ☐ Formula ☐ _____ Cal

Caregiving Interval _Q4_

Feeding Interval _IV LIPIDS & HYPERALIMENT._

Other _____

Current Issues and Concerns: _____

1. _PDA_

2. _OXYGENATION_

3. _HYPERBILIRUBINEMIA_

4. _ENERGY_

Current Medical Problems:

Pneumothorax	☐	Tracheostomy	☐
Hypoglycemia	☐	Hypoxic Events	☐
Hyperbilirubinemia	☒	Acidosis: pH<7.3	☐
Hydrocephalus	☐	Hypotension	☐
NEC ☐ PDA	☒	Feeding Difficulty	☐
Renal ☐ Sepsis ☐		Bleeding Tendency	☐
Seizures	☐	Anemia ☐ Apnea	☐
Bradycardia	☐	# Episodes/Day____	

Page 1

ankles and feet pointed outward into the blanket roll. He wore a diaper, which appeared big for him. Robert had his right arm tucked up close to his right shoulder, his hand tightly fisted. His stretched out left arm had an IV line going to his wrist. His left hand was also tightly fisted. Leads to keep track of his heart rate, breathing rate, the oxygen level in his blood stream, and his body temperature were fastened to his chest, back, and left foot. The lines attached to him were draped alongside him.

CURRENT OBSERVATION CIRCUMSTANCES

Location: Fullterm nursery ☐   Isolation Rm. ☐   Intermediate ☐   NICU ☒

         NICU Parent Rm. ☐   Parent's Room ☐   Home ☐   Other _____

Environment: Table ☐   Open Crib ☐   Incubator ☒   Mock Crib ☐

         Other _____

Bedding, Clothing, and Other Facilitation:

Mattress ☒	Hammock ☐	Waterbed ☐		
Bunting ☐	Clothing ☐	Water Glove ☐		
Hat ☐	Pacifier ☐	Side rolls/Foot rolls ☒	*"NESTER" WITH STRAPS:*	*SOME SOFT BEDDING UNDER BEDROLL*
Sheepskin:	Natural ☐	Synthetic ☒		
Blanket:	Loose ☐	Secure ☐	Tight ☐	
Incubator/crib cover:	Partial ☐	Thin/Light ☐	Thick/Dark ☐	
Personal Items:	Pictures ☐	Photos ☒	Decals ☐	Stuffed Animals ☒ x

Others: _____ *SISTER + BROTHER*

CLOTH DIAPER UNDER HEAD; DIAPER; BILIMASK; IV in LEFT ARM; LEADS: TEMP, HR, RR, Sa O$_2$

Ambient Light, Sound, and Activity Levels:

Sound: 1 2 3 4 5 6 7 ⑧ 9
1 is very quiet as if in a closed door parent room without interruption
9 is very loud, for instance with radio on high volume, staff voices, telephone ringing and monitors sounding
Describe: *HI FI VENTILATOR; VOICES; ALARMS; INFANTS CRYING; REFUSE RECEPTACLES; EQUIPMENT; PAPERS; FOOTSTEPS; INCUBATOR NEXT TO OPEN DOOR*

Light: 1 2 3 4 5 6 7 8 ⑨
1 is a semi-dark room, shielded incubator, no overhead lights;
9 is bright overhead and/or side lights, no covering on crib or incubator
Describe: *BILIRUBIN LIGHTS; BRIGHT SUNSHINE - BLINDING TO STAFF (SHIELDING THEIR EYES) BRIGHT OVERHEAD LIGHTS ON*

Activity: 1 2 3 4 5 6 7 ⑧ 9
1 is very calm, quiet, soothing or no activity around the baby, e.g. no staff movement, or very soft, unhurried walking, etc.
9 is hectic, continuously changing activity, with visitors, staff, x-ray machine, personnel hurrying about, water running, equipment being moved, etc.
Describe: *MUCH STAFF MOVEMENT; PARENTS; INTERRUPTION OF BEDSIDE NURSE BY OTHER NURSE*

Caregiver(s) Observed: Physician ☐   Nurse ☒   Parent ☐   OT/PT ☐   Other _____

Caregiving Actions Observed: (list in chronological sequence) *ARRANGEMENT OF MATERIALS; BILILIGHTS OFF; ATTENDS TO OTHER NURSE; OBSERVATION; IMMEDIATE TEMP-TAKING; POSITION CHANGE TO SUPINE; STETHOSCOPE; DIAPER CHANGE; LISTENING TO PULSE; CORD CARE; POSITION CHANGE TO PRONE; "NESTER" ADJUSTMENT; BILIRUBIN LIGHTS TURNED ON AGAIN.*

Time and Duration of Observation:

interaction ____ *14*
interaction ____ *8*
interaction ____ *18*
40

3. Robert's Behavior during Observation before Caregiving Interaction
Robert was observed for about 14 minutes before his nurse stepped to his bedside. He appeared to be lying there very quietly, perhaps sleeping. The fisting of his hands at times became even tighter. He was pale and appeared quite yellow; his legs and feet were very dark and dusky. He breathed with fluttering breaths, at times quite shallow and labored, at other times fast and unsteady, with approximately 30–40 breaths a minute. His heart rate was quite steady with about 130–140 beats per minute. The

NIDCAP behavioral observation sheets for Robert A.

OBSERVATION SHEET Name: *ROBERT A.* Date: *1 MARCH 1995* Sheet Number *1*

LAUGHTER / VOICES WALKING CRYING

		Time: 12 / 8 (0-2)	14 (3-4)	16 (5-6)	18 (7-8)	20 (9-10)			Time: 12 / 8 (0-2)	14 (3-4)	16 (5-6)	18 (7-8)	20 (9-10)
Resp:	Regular						**State:** 1A						
	Irregular	✓	✓	✓	✓	✓	1B						
	Slow		✓	✓FL	✓FL	✓FL	2A ? [FL=FLUTTERING]	✓	✓	✓	✓	✓	
	Fast	FL	✓✓	✓FL	✓		2B						
	Pause						UNDER 3A						
Color:	Jaundice	✓	✓	✓	✓	✓	BILIRUBIN 3B						
	Pink						LIGHTS 4A						
	Pale	✓	✓	✓	✓	✓	& WITH 4B						
	Webb						MASKED 5A						
	Red						EYES 5B						
	Dusky FEET↑	✓	✓	✓	✓✓	✓	6A						
	Blue						6B						
	Tremor						AA						
	Startle						**Face** Mouthing						✓✓
	Twitch Face					✓	(cont.): Suck Search						
	Twitch Body			✓			Sucking						
	Twitch Extremities						**Extrem.:** Finger Splay						
Visceral/ Resp:	Spit up						Airplane						
	Gag						Salute						
	Burp						Sitting On Air						
	Hiccough						Hand Clasp						
	BM Grunt						Foot Clasp						
	Sounds						Hand to Mouth						
	Sigh		✓	✓			Grasping		✓✓	✓	✓	✓	
	Gasp						Holding On		✓	✓	✓	✓	
Motor:	Flaccid Arm(s)	✓	✓	✓	✓	✓	Fisting	P✓	✓P✓	P✓	P✓	P	
	Flaccid leg(s)						**Attention:** Fuss						
	Flexed/Tucked Arms Act. Post.	✓	✓	✓	✓	✓	Yawn						
	Flexed/Tucked Legs Act. Post.	✓	✓	✓	✓	✓	Sneeze						
	Extend Arms Act. Post.	✓✓					Face Open						
	Extend Legs Act. Post.						Eye Floating						
	Smooth Mvmt Arms						Avert						
	Smooth Mvmt Legs						Frown						
	Smooth Mvmt Trunk						Ooh Face						
	Stretch/Drown						Locking						
	Diffuse Squirm						Cooing						
	Arch						Speech Mvmt.						
	Tuck Trunk						**Posture:** (Prone, Supine, Side)	PRONE	→	→	→	→	
	Leg Brace						**Head:** (Right, Left, Middle)	L	→	→	→	→	
Face:	Tongue Extension						**Location:** (Crib, Isolette, Held)	INCUB	→	→	→	→	
	Hand on Face						**Manipulation:**	—	—	—	—	—	
	Gape Face						Heart Rate	129	136	133	137	133	
	Grimace						Respiration Rate	46	48	40	42	34	
	Smile						TcPO₂ / SaO₂ →	99	99	100	76/80	100	

2002 02 1M (12/83) HAis 1981

oxygen level in his bloodstream stayed steady much of the time at about 99%, with only one dip to 76% after his breathing had become quite irregular for a period. As he squirmed and adjusted his position, he recovered his oxygen level quickly.

4. Robert's Behavior during Caregiving Interaction

   As Robert's nurse stepped to his bedside, she first arranged the necessary

OBSERVATION SHEET　Name: *ROBERT A.*　　Date: *1 MARCH 1995*　Sheet Number *2*　ALARMS
STAFF WALKING, ALARMS VOICES

Category	Item	22 / 8 (0-2)	24 (3-4)	26 (5-6)	28 (7-8)	30 (9-10)
Resp:	Regular					
	Irregular	✓	✓	✓	✓	✓
	Slow					
	Fast	✓	✓	✓	✓	✓
	Pause	FL.	✓	FL.	✓	✓
Color:	Jaundice	✓✓	✓	✓	✓	✓✓
	Pink					
	Pale	✓	✓			
	Webb					
	Red					✓✓✓
	Dusky	✓	✓	✓✓	✓✓✓	✓✓✓
	Blue					
	Tremor					
	Startle					
	Twitch Face					
	Twitch Body			✓		
	Twitch Extremities					
Visceral/ Resp:	Spit up					
	Gag					
	Burp					
	Hiccough					
	BM Grunt					
	Sounds					
	Sigh					
	Gasp					
Motor:	Flaccid Arm(s)					
	Flaccid leg(s)					
	Flexed/Tucked Arms Act.	✓	✓	✓	✓	✓
	Flexed/Tucked Arms Post.					✓✓
	Flexed/Tucked Legs Act.	✓	✓	✓	✓	✓✓✓
	Flexed/Tucked Legs Post.			✓		✓✓
	Extend Arms Act./Post.					✓
	Extend Legs Act./Post.					✓
	Smooth Mvmt Arms					
	Smooth Mvmt Legs					
	Smooth Mvmt Trunk					
	Stretch/Drown					
	Diffuse Squirm					✓
	Arch					
	Tuck Trunk			✓		✓✓
	Leg Brace				✓	✓✓
Face:	Tongue Extension					
	Hand on Face					
	Gape Face					
	Grimace					
	Smile					

(UNDER BILILIGHTS & WITH MASK) — annotation at State 2A
FLAILING — annotation at left Motor section

Category	Item	22 / 8 (0-2)	24 (3-4)	26 (5-6)	28 (7-8)	30 (9-10)
State:	1A					
	1B					
	2A	✓	✓	✓	✓	✓
	2B					
	3A					
	3B					
	4A					
	4B					CRYFACE
	5A					✓
	5B					
	6A					✓
	6B					
	AA					
Face (cont.):	Mouthing					✓
	Suck Search					
	Sucking					
Extrem.:	Finger Splay					
	Airplane					✓✓
	Salute					
	Sitting On Air					
	Hand Clasp					
	Foot Clasp					
	Hand to Mouth					
	Grasping	✓		✓	✓	✓✓
	Holding On				✓✓	✓
	Fisting	✓	✓		✓✓	
Attention:	Fuss					
	Yawn					
	Sneeze					
	Face Open					
	Eye Floating					
	Avert					
	Frown					
	Ooh Face	✓	✓			
	Locking					
	Cooing					
	Speech Mvmt.					
Posture:	(Prone, Supine, Side)	PR→	→	SUPINE→		→
Head:	(Right, Left, Middle)	L	→	→R	→	→
Location:	(Crib, Isolette, Held)	INCUB.	→	→	→	→
Manipulation:		—	—	LIGHTS OBSERVE	POSITION CHANGE HR CRED	LEAVES PTINES
	Heart Rate	141	140	147	153	162
	Respiration Rate	32	48	38	?	?
	TcPO₂ / SaO₂	98	97	99	94	96/89

materials for the planned caregiving interaction, then she observed Robert for a minute counting his breathing ratc. She turned off the bilirubin light above him and moved it away from the bedside, opened the portholes of the incubator, and placed a thermometer under Robert's left arm. Robert immediately became dark and dusky and quickly pulled his arms closer in, fisting more tightly and pulling his legs up. The oxygen level in his bloodstream dropped to 88% and he paused in his breathing. His nurse turned

OBSERVATION SHEET Name: _ROBERT A._ Date: _1 MARCH 1995_ Sheet Number _3_

PAPER VOICES↑ TEL. EQUIP. ALARMS

	Time:	32 / 0-2	34 / 3-4	36 / 5-6	38 / 7-8	40 / 9-10
Resp:	Regular					
	Irregular	✓	✓	✓	✓	✓
	Slow					
	Fast					
	Pause	✓	✓	✓	✓	✓
Color:	Jaundice	✓	✓			
	Pink					
	Pale		✓			
	Webb					
	Red	✓	✓			
	Dusky		✓✓	✓	✓✓✓	✓✓✓
	Blue					
	Tremor					
	Startle					
	Twitch Face					
	Twitch Body			✓	✓✓	✓
	Twitch Extremities					
Visceral/ Resp:	Spit up					
	Gag					
	Burp					
	Hiccough					
	BM Grunt					
	Sounds					
	Sigh					
	Gasp					
Motor:	Flaccid Arm(s)					
	Flaccid leg(s)					
	Flexed/Tucked Arms Act./Post.					
	Flexed/Tucked Legs Act./Post.					
	Extend Arms Act./Post.					
	Extend Legs Act./Post.					
	Smooth Mvmt Arms					
	Smooth Mvmt Legs					
	Smooth Mvmt Trunk					
	Stretch/Drown					
	Diffuse Squirm					
	Arch					
	Tuck Trunk					
	Leg Brace					
Face:	Tongue Extension					
	Hand on Face					
	Gape Face					
	Grimace					
	Smile					

	Time:	32 / 0-2	34 / 3-4	36 / 5-6	38 / 7-8	40 / 9-10
State:	1A					
	1B					
(UNDER	2A	✓				
BILILIGHT	2B					
& MASK)	3A ?	✓	✓	✓	✓	✓
	3B					
	4A	✓?	✓?			
	4B					
	5A					
	5B					
	6A					
	6B					
	AA					
Face (cont.):	Mouthing	✓	✓✓	✓✓	✓	✓
	Suck Search					
	Sucking					
Extrem.:	Finger Splay					
	Airplane					
	Salute					
	Sitting On Air					
	Hand Clasp					
	Foot Clasp					
	Hand to Mouth			✓✓	✓	
	Grasping					
	Holding On					
	Fisting					
Attention:	Fuss					
	Yawn					
	Sneeze					
	Face Open	✓	✓✓	✓	✓	✓
	Eye Floating					
	Avert					
	Frown					
	Ooh Face					
	Locking					
	Cooing					
	Speech Mvmt.					
Posture:	(Prone, Supine, Side)	SUP PRONE →	→	→	→	
Head:	(Right, Left, Middle)	R→L	L	L	L	L
Location:	(Crib, Isolette, Held)	INCUB.	→	→	→	→
Manipulation:	TURN LIGHT ON / POSITION ON		—	—	—	
	Heart Rate	157	128	125	134	132
	Respiration Rate	?	26	26	?	40
	TcPO₂ / SaO₂ →		75	92	98/89	94/87

2002 02 1M (12/83) H Als 1981

him onto his back, one hand under his buttocks and one under his shoulders; Robert's arms flew out to the side, fingers completely extended. He attempted to bring his arms back in and tuck his legs and feet in, turning his ankles outward into the bedding and grasping with his toes and fingers. His nurse now listened to his chest and belly and took his pulse with a stethoscope. She then pulled her hands out of the incubator and attended to another staff member who had come to her with a question. Robert's

OBSERVATION SHEET Name: ROBERT A. Date: 1 MARCH 1995 Sheet Number 4

Right-side time header annotation: ALARMS ALARMS ALARMS VOICES↑ALARMS

Left annotation on State rows: (UNDER BILILIGHT AND WITH MASK)

		42 8 / 0-2	44 / 3-4	46 / 5-6	48 / 7-8	50 / 9-10
Resp:	Regular					
	Irregular	✓	✓	✓	✓	✓
	Slow	✓	✓	✓ FL	(✓) FL	✓ FL
	Fast					
	Pause	✓	✓	✓	✓	
Color:	Jaundice	✓	✓	✓		✓
	Pink					
	Pale					
	Webb					
	Red					
	Dusky FEET↑	✓✓	✓✓	✓✓✓	✓✓✓	✓✓✓
	Blue					
	Tremor					
	Startle					
	Twitch Face					
	Twitch Body			✓	✓✓✓	
	Twitch Extremities					
Visceral/ Resp:	Spit up					
	Gag					
	Burp					
	Hiccough					
	BM Grunt					
	Sounds					
	Sigh					
	Gasp					
Motor:	Flaccid Arm(s) TRUNK		→	→	→	
	Flaccid leg(s)					
	Flexed/Tucked Arms Act. Post.	✓	✓	✓	✓	✓
	Flexed/Tucked Legs Act. Post.	✓	✓	✓	✓	✓
	Extend Arms Act. Post.					
	Extend Legs Act. Post.					
	Smooth Mvmt Arms					
	Smooth Mvmt Legs					
	Smooth Mvmt Trunk					
	Stretch/Drown					
	Diffuse Squirm	✓	✓			
	Arch					
	Tuck Trunk		✓			
	Leg Brace	✓P	✓P	✓P	✓P	✓P
Face:	Tongue Extension					
	Hand on Face					
	Gape Face					
	Grimace					
	Smile					

		42 8 / 0-2	44 / 3-4	46 / 5-6	48 / 7-8	50 / 9-10
State:	1A					
	1B					
	2A	✓?	✓	✓?	✓	✓
	2B					
	3A	✓?	✓			
	3B					
	4A					
	4B					
	5A					
	5B					
	6A					
	6B					
	AA					
Face (cont.):	Mouthing	✓	✓	✓✓	✓	✓
	Suck Search					
	Sucking					
Extrem.:	Finger Splay					
	Airplane					
	Salute					
	Sitting On Air					
	Hand Clasp					
	Foot Clasp					
	Hand to Mouth	✓	✓	✓P	✓P	✓P
	Grasping					
	Holding On					
	Fisting	✓P				
Attention:	Fuss					
	Yawn					
	Sneeze					
	Face Open					
	Eye Floating					
	Avert					
	Frown					
	Ooh Face					
	Locking					
	Cooing					
	Speech Mvmt.					
Posture:	(Prone, Supine, Side)	PRONE	→	→	→	→
Head:	(Right, Left, Middle)	L	→	→	→	→
Location:	(Crib, Isolette, Held)	INCUBATOR	→	→	→	→
Manipulation:		—	—	—	—	—
	Heart Rate	129	141	135	137	144
	Respiration Rate	44	44	38	34	32
	TcPO₂/SaO₂	95	94	96	95	95

2002 02 1M (12/83) H-Als 1981

breathing was still quite unsteady. He continued to make efforts to tuck his arms closer in and grasp, reaching with his hands and feet. His face puckered up and his forehead furrowed, and he appeared to cry. His oxygen level dropped to 89% as his heart rate rose to 162 beats per minute. He became increasingly dark and dusky all over, his feet now deep purple. His nurse gathered Robert up, briefly holding him in, and then turned him quickly onto his tummy facing to his left, his head elevated on a folded diaper, his neck and shoulders sinking off the diaper. She adjusted the blanket rolls around him and fastened several straps across his back, holding the nest's edges together. Then she closed the incubator doors and moved the bilirubin lights back into position, turning them on above Robert. Robert attempted to settle, tucking his arms close up to his chest, with his knees and ankles turned out. The inside of his feet pressed into his bedding. He was very dark and dusky, breathed irregularly, and appeared to be awake, his eyebrows raised above the bili-mask and his mouth opening and closing as if searching.

5. Robert's Behavior following Caregiving Interaction

   For the next 6 minutes Robert squirmed and attempted to tuck himself more together, twitching and searching with his mouth. He brought his left hand closer up to his mouth, one finger touching his lips. His eyebrows and forehead were raised, and he was probably awake under his mask. During the course of these efforts, the oxygen level in Robert's bloodstream repeatedly dropped below 85%. Each time he recovered with further squirming. Gradually his face appeared to lose energy and he became very still. His shoulders sank more into the bedding. His left hand stayed close to his mouth and occasionally his mouth opened and closed slightly. He was quite dark and purple, his heart rate between 130 and 145 beats per minute. His breathing fluttered and at times was quite labored with an overall rate between 30 and 46 breaths per minute. The oxygen level in his bloodstream now remained relatively steady at 95%. He appeared to be quite exhausted.

Summary

Robert was born at 29 weeks of pregnancy to his 31-year-old mother, who has two other children. Mrs. A's pregnancy was complicated by high blood pressure. At 28 weeks, she had some vaginal bleeding and contractions. She was admitted to the hospital for 4 days and given medication (dexamethasone) in support of Robert's lung maturation, and medication (terbutaline) to help prevent premature delivery. Mrs. A continued the terbutaline treatment at home for 4 more days, when labor began. On her way to the regional maternity hospital, St. L., Robert's father stopped at a hospital nearer to the parents' home since Robert was ready to be born, feet first. He was somewhat limp at birth with poor color, as reflected in his score of well-being (Apgar Score) of 5 out of 10 at 1 minute, 10 being the best score. He recovered quickly and by 5 minutes was given a score of 7, by 10 minutes a score of 9. He was given oxygen and transported together with his mother to St. L. Hospital. At birth, Robert weighed 2 lbs, 15 oz (1340 g; 50%ile), measured 15 inches (38 cm; 50%ile), with a head circumference of 11 inches (28 cm; 75%ile). This shows that he had grown appropriately in his mother's womb. Once in the intensive care nursery, Robert's breathing was supported with oxygen for less than a day. Since then he has been breathing room air on his own, supported with some medication (caffeine). A vessel in his heart that was open in the womb continues to be open (patent ductus arteriosus; PDA). To support its closing, Robert receives steroid medication (Indocin). In order to protect his intestines from bleeding, his feeding has been stopped for the time being and he receives fluids by IV. Robert is now 4 days old and has developed jaundice, which is treated with special light therapy (phototherapy; bilirubin lights). From the observation, Robert appears to be a competent and very sensitive infant. He makes repeated efforts to adjust his position in the incubator to be more comfortable. When cared for, he makes strong efforts to tuck himself together and to settle himself. Despite the mask covering his eyes, he makes great efforts to look. He also attempts to find something to suck on. He brings his hands to his mouth quite readily. His sensitivity shows itself in his color changes, his shallow and labored breathing, the occasional drops in oxygen level and his increasing exhaustion.

Robert's Current Goals

From the observation Robert appears to be working towards:

1. Becoming increasingly robust and steady in his breathing and oxygen levels when resting and when interacted with.
2. Becoming increasingly successful in pulling himself into a more tucked restful position, bringing his hands to his mouth and bracing his legs into his bedding.
3. Awakening and looking, as well as sucking.

Recommendations

In support of Robert's goal strivings, the following suggestions may be helpful:

1. Nursery Environment
   a. Consider exploring opportunities to reduce the sound generated by staff voices, alarms, the respirator at the next bedside, telephones, etc.
   b. In support of a calmer environment, consider reducing the light levels in the room by drawing the blinds when the sunlight is bright, and by reducing overhead lighting.
   c. Consider providing a darkened environment throughout the day for Robert in support of his alerting and sleep development; consider the use of a specialized light therapy blanket (biliblanket), which will free-up his eyes from needing to be patched.
   d. Consider rearranging the cabinets at the foot of the beds in order to reduce the congestion in the room.
   e. Consider keeping the room door closed in order to reduce sound from the hallway.
2. Bedspace and Bedding
   a. Consider developing an inviting atmosphere around Robert's bedspace for his parents, brother, and sister to be with him for extended periods as well as in support of the comfort of his professional caregivers.
   b. Consider a reclining chair supportive of Robert's parents and professional caregivers when holding Robert wrapped in a bilirubin blanket without eye patches, thereby facilitating his strengths, energy, and opportunity to look.

      c. Consider providing Robert with a soft, well-aligned nest, perhaps bedding him lying on his side, and giving him the opportunity to tuck into a contained restful position.

      d. Consider using a very small diaper for Robert in support of a more well-aligned position for his legs.

      e. Consider bedding Robert with a long soft pillow to hug with his arms and legs, bringing his knees and ankles together when lying on his side.

3. Caregiving Interaction

      a. Consider Robert as an active partner in his care and as a competent child who makes strong efforts to be restful and tucked together.

      b. Consider using your observation of Robert's breathing rate at the beginning of your caregiving interaction as an opportunity to let Robert tell you what he is attempting to accomplish.

      c. Consider removing Robert's eye patches when you care for and interact with him; observe his reaction and give him an opportunity to relax and recover from the periods of eye patching; give him the opportunity to experience and enjoy the social interchange with you.

      d. Consider introducing your hands to Robert first, learn how he responds to you and assist him in accomplishing the position and actions he is aiming for, before you engage in specific caregiving tasks.

      e. Consider supporting Robert gently into lying on his side; encourage him to hold onto your hands and offer him opportunities to suck. Contain him while taking his vital signs and changing his diaper.

      f. Consider containing and holding Robert when you interact with him; give him the opportunity to experience smooth movements of his arms and legs.

      g. Consider involving a physical or occupational therapist in Robert's care in order to evaluate his leg and foot position, as well as to consult you about the best ways to support his leg position and movement.

      h. Consider seeking developmental guidance in caring for Robert and in supporting your caregiving interactions to become increasingly collaborative with Robert. Enjoy his competence and your facilitation of his efforts.

APPENDIX B: BEHAVIORAL DEFINITIONS (Derived from Als, 1981)

The behaviors observed are organized into Autonomic/Visceral, State, Motor, and Attention-Related behavior groups.

Autonomic Behaviors

Respiration

These are subgrouped into respiration patterns, colors, autonomic instability-related motor patterns, and visceral and specific respiratory patterns.

Regular: The breath-to-breath interval is steady.

Irregular: The breath-to-breath interval is variable, at times short, at times longer.

Slow: Less than at a comparable rate of 40 respirations/minute.

Fast: More than at a comparable rate of 60 respirations/minute.

Pause: Any cessation of respiration for equal to or longer than 2 seconds.

More than one category can be checked, e.g., regular and slow or irregular and slow and fast, and/or pause.

Color

Jaundice: Yellowish appearance; yellowness of skin and whites of eyes.

Pink: Good perfusion with pink coloring throughout the face, including perioral and temple area; if trunk and extremities are observable, the same criteria apply.

Pale: Whitish, sallow appearance in parts of face, e.g., forehead, perinasal or oral area, temples or overall skin color appearance. Gray, although one hopes it is not observed, would be noted with a special comment under pale.

Webbed: Pattern of surface blood vessels visible in the form of a net or webb, often in face, neck, at times total body surface including extremities.

Red: Overly perfused, plethoric-appearing coloration.

Dusky: Purple, dark hue of face, parts of the face, or body surface.

Blue: Cyanotic, pale in perioral, other areas of the face, trunk, or extremities. More than one color category may be appropriate to mark either because of temporal fluctuations or because patches of various colors are observed (e.g., pale and blue or dusky and webbed, etc.). Notes as to special circumstances such as harlequin pattern should be made.

Autonomic Instability-Related Motor Patterns

Tremor: Trembling or quivering of any part of or of whole body, e.g., leg tremor, chin tremor.

Startle: Sudden large amplitude jumping movement of arms or trunk or legs or whole body.

Twitch (face, body, extremities): Small amplitude, brief contractile response of a skeletal muscle elicited, presumably by a single maximal volley of impulses in the neurons supplying it; marked as to the location of its occurrence.

Visceral and Respiratory Behaviors

Spit up: Any bringing up of feeding or saliva; more than a drool is required.

Gag: The infant appears to choke momentarily or gulp; the respiratory pattern is disrupted during a gag. Gags are often but not necessarily accompanied by mild mouth opening.

Burp: The infant brings up air in an expiratory burst.

Hiccough: The infant hiccoughs, i.e., makes one or repetitive sharp inspiratory sounds with spasm of the glottis and diaphragm.

BM Grunt: Bowel movement grunting or straining. The infant's face and body display the straining often associated with bowel movements and/or the infant emits the grunting sounds often associated with bowel movements and/or actually passes gas or defecates.

Sounds: The infants emits undifferentiated whimperlike sounds that resemble involuntary vocal discharges.

Sigh: The infant in-and exhales, perhaps audibly, in a breath longer and deeper than his current respiratory pattern.

Gasp: The infant draws in a respiration sharply or laboriously, often after a respiratory pause; the infant may not apparently complete the inspiration and does not move smoothly to the next expiration.

Motor System Behaviors

These are subgrouped into general extremity and trunk behaviors, specific extremity behavior, and behaviors of the face.

General Extremity and Trunk Behaviors

Flaccid arm(s): The tone of one or both arms is very low and the arm(s) are lying flaccidly or are held limply. Flexor or extensor postural adjustment may be observed in the presence of flaccidity.

Flaccid leg(s): The tone of one or both legs is very low and the leg(s) are lying or are held flaccidly or limply. Again, flexor or extensor postural adjustment may be observed in the presence of flaccidity. Note: It is very important to differentiate relaxation from flaccidity. The easiest way to learn to distinguish the two qualities of muscle tone is to test the relative activity of tone by lifting the limb in question. If tone is flaccid, a droopy, limp reaction and lack of response will be felt; if tone is active, a self-maintained tonic response will be felt.

Flexed or Tucked Arm(s): Act: Activity
                        Post: Posture
Activity: Refers to the current flexor movement or act of tucking in of the arm(s). This may be repetitive activity or one adjustment.
Posture: Refers to the maintenance of arm(s) in a flexor position.

Flexed or Tucked Legs(s): Act: Activity
                        Post: Posture
Activity: Refers to the active flexor movement or tucking movement of the leg(s), whether it is then maintained or not. It can be repetitive flexor adjustments
Posture: Refers to the maintenance of the leg(s) in a flexor or tucked position.

Extend Arm(s): Act: Activity
                Post: Posture

Activity: Refers to the active extension movement of one or both arms. This may be a single or several consecutive actions, often alternating with some flexor movement, in which case both *extend act* and *flex act* are marked.

Posture: Refers to the maintenance of arm(s) in extension either in midair or on a surface.

Extend Leg(s): Act: Activity
                  Post: Posture

Activity: Refers to the active extension movement of one or both legs. This may be a single or several consecutive actions, often alternating with some flexor movement, in which case both *extend act* and *flex act* would be marked.

Posture: Refers to the maintenance of legs in extension either in midair or on a surface.

Sm Mvmt Arms: Smooth movement of arms

Sm Mvmt Legs: Smooth movement of legs

Sm Mvmt Trunk Smooth movement of trunk

Refers to smooth movement of arms, legs, or trunk, balanced in terms of extensor and flexor component and showing apparent control by the infant.

Stretch/Drown: This is a configuration of labored trunkal extension, often also accompanied by arm extension and at times leg extension, which is then followed by an apparent effort to move the trunk back into flexion. This pattern of stretching and tucking may be repeated several times. At times the stretching component is quite prolonged. It frequently follows a pattern of decreasing respiratory rate at times ending in a respiratory pause. Often in the course of this motor pattern, inspiration or expiration has halted, leading to increasing color change. The pattern gives the impression of the struggling action of drowning, while attempting to regain breathing. It is also referred to as "motor drown." Care needs to be given to the successful reactivation of respiration. In successful efforts after a burst of drowning-like behavior, respiration restarts, albeit now often tachypneically. In other cases the drowning may be followed by limpness and a prolonged respiratory pause, requiring stimulation or at least containment into successful trunkal and extremity flexion.

Diffuse Squirm: Refers to small writhing, wriggling motions of the trunk, often with accompanying movements of the extremities, yet not showing the labored stretching, struggling patterns of *stretch/drown*. At times, however, *diff squirm* may lead to *stretch/drown*.

Arch: Refers to trunkal arching or trunkal extension into an arch and/or head extension, in prone, supine, or upright position. The upper extremities may or may not extend; the legs often may extend.

Tuck Trunk: This refers to trunkal flexion activity or maintained flexor posture. The infant curls or tucks trunk and/or shoulders into flexion; often the infant may pull the legs up into flexion or pull the arms in simultaneously. Active trunkal flexion movement in prone, supine, side-lying, or sitting position as well as the maintenance of trunkally flexed posture are marked.

Leg Brace The infant extends leg(s) and/or feet towards the edge or wall of the isoletts, crib, etc., or the caregiver's hand or body, as if in an effort to stabilize and gain boundary and inhibition to extensor movement or posture. Once touching, the infant may flex the legs and relax while maintaining the bracing, or may restart the active bracing efforts. Even if no surface is available against which the bracing can be successful, efforts at apparently seeking such a surface should be marked in this category. The infant may be actively pressing one or both feet against the mattress or a blanket roll, etc.

Face Behaviors

Tongue Extension: The infant's tongue protrudes in extension beyond the lips or extends encased in the lower lip. The behavior is marked whether the infant maintains this tongue posture or engages in repeated extension and flexion or relaxation movements of the tongue. Soft modulated speech-like tongue movements or mouthing are not marked in this category.

Hand on Face: The infant's hand or hands are placed onto the face or over the ears and are maintained there for at least a brief or for a prolonged period. The movement is distinguished from active grasping. It is a more protective, occluding-appearing, usually soft movement that creates a barrier between the face and the outside world. The hand may be placed palm down or palm up against the face.

Gape Face: This refers to a drooping open mouth configuration that is the result of decreased lower facial tone. It gives the appearance of exhaustion and facial limpness. It may be paired, however, with eyes open and even environment inspection. It is also seen in sleep.

Grimace: This is a facial extension configuration often accompanied by lip retraction and facial retraction and distortion. Eyebrow knitting or frowning is not typically a part of this configuration, since it represents facial flexion rather than facial extension.

Smile: Smiling requires facial relaxation without flaccidity and is formed by an at least slightly upward curving of the corner(s) of the mouth, often accompanied by a momentary or prolonged softening of the cheeks.

Mouthing: The infant makes one or repetitive lip and/or jaw opening and closing movements. These are distinguished from suck-searching. In mouthing, the lips stay usually soft and relaxed and are not directed forward.

Suck Search: The infant actively extends the lips forward or sideways and/or opens the mouth in a searching, rooting fashion; the infant often moves the head while doing so, as if to find something to suck on.

Sucking: The infant sucks on the hand or fingers, on clothing, bedding, the caregiver's finger or breast, a pacifier or other object that the infant has either obtained or that the caregiver has inserted into the infant's mouth.

Specific Extremity Movements

Finger Splay: The infant's hand(s) open and the fingers are extended and separated from each other.

Airplane: The infant's arm(s) are either fully extended out to the side at approximately shoulder level or upper and lower arm are at an angle to each other and are extended out at the shoulder.

Salute: The infant's arm(s) are fully extended into mid air, either singly or simultaneously. This is often but not necessarily accompanied by finger splaying.

Sitting on Air: The infant's legs are extended into mid air either singly or simultaneously. This may occur in supine, side-lying, or in upright position.

Hand Clasp: The infant grasps the hands or clutches the hands midline to the body. The hands each may be closed but they hold onto each other or actively press against each other. Interdigitation of fingers of one hand with those of the other hand is a subcategory of hand clasp and is marked here.

Foot Clasp: The infant positions one foot against the other, either foot sole to foot sole or one foot sole against the other leg, or he folds the legs in a crossed position with feet grasping the legs or resting against them.

Hand to Mouth: The infant attempts to bring hands or fingers to the mouth in an apparent effort to suck on them. The effort does not have to be successful to be marked.

Grasping: The infant makes grasping movements with the hands, either directed at the face or body, or in midair, or to the caregiver's hands or fingers or body, the infant's own bottle, tubing or bedding, the side of the bassinet, etc.

Holding On: Holding on to the examiner's hands or finger or arm, etc., with the infant's own hands; the infant may have placed them there, or the examiner may have positioned them there; the infant then actively holds on.

Fisting: The infant appears to hold on to the infant's own hand by flexing the fingers and forming a fist. Occasionally fisting is observed with an object in hand (e.g., the edge of a blanket, etc.). The tightness of the flexion differentiates the softer holding on from fisting.

State-Related Behaviors

These are subgrouped into the states themselves and specific, typically attention-related behaviors. Various configurations of behaviors encompassing eye movements, eye opening and facial expressions, gross body movements, respirations, and tonus aspects are used in specific temporal relationships to one another to determine at what level of consciousness an infant is at a particular time. It is possible to make meaningful, systematic distinctions between dynamic transformations of various behavioral configurations that appear to correspond to varying states of availability and conscious responsiveness. The following spectrum of observable states is suggested: states labeled as A states are "noisy," unclean, and diffuse; states labeled as B states are clean, well-defined states.

Sleep States

State 1A: Infant in deep sleep with obligatory regular breathing or breathing in synchrony with only the respirator, eyes closed, no eye movements under closed lids; quiet facial expression; no spontaneous activity; typically poor color.

State 1B: Infant in deep sleep with predominantly modulated regular breathing; eyes closed, no eye movements under closed lids, relaxed facial expression; no spontaneous activity except isolated startles.

State 2A: Light sleep with eyes closed, rapid eye movements can be observed under closed lids; low amplitude activity level with diffuse and disorganized movements; respirations are irregular and there are many sucking and mouthing movements, whimpers; facial, body, and extremity twitchings, much grimacing; the impression of a "noisy" state is given. Color is typically poor.

State 2B: Light sleep with eyes closed; rapid eye movements can be observed under closed lids; low activity level with movements and dampened startles; movements are likely to be of lower amplitude and more monitored than in state 1; infant responds to various internal stimuli with dampened startle. Respirations are more regular, mild sucking and mouthing movements can occur off and on; one or two whimpers may be observed, as well as infrequent sighs or smiles.

Transitional (Drowsy) States

State 3A: Drowsy or semi-dozing; eyes may be open or closed, eyelids fluttering or exaggerated blinking; if eyes open, glassy veiled look; activity level variable, with or without interspersed, startles from time to time; diffuse movement; fussing and/or much discharge of vocalization, whimpers, facial grimacing, etc.

State 3B: Drowsy, same as above but with less discharge of vocalization, whimpers, facial grimacing, etc.

Awake States

In the box 4A, two types of diffuse alertness are distinguished, 4AL and 4AH. L or H is marked instead of a check mark.

State 4AL: Awake and quiet, minimal motor activity, eyes half open or open but with glazed or dull look, giving the impression of little involvement and distance; or focused yet seeming to look through, rather than at, object or examiner; or the infant is clearly awake and reactive but has his eyes closed intermittently.

State 4AH: Awake and quiet, minimal motor activity, eyes wide open, "hyperalert" or giving the impression of panic or fear; may appear to be hooked by the stimulus; seems to have difficulty in modulating or breaking the intensity of the fixation to the object or move away from it.

State 4B: Alert with bright shiny animated facial expression; seems to focus attention on source of stimulation and appears to process information actively and with modulation; motor activity is at a minimum.

Active States

State 5A: Eyes may or may not be open but infant is clearly awake and aroused, as indicated by motor arousal, tonus, and distressed facial expression, grimacing, or other signs of discomfort. Fussing, if present, is diffuse or strained.

State 5B: Eyes may or may not be open but infant is clearly awake and aroused, with considerable, yet well-defined, motor activity. Infant may also be clearly fussing but not crying robustly.

Crying States

State 6A: Intense crying, as indicated by intense grimace and cry face, yet cry sound may be very strained or very weak or absent; intensity of upset is greater than fussing.

State 6B: Rhythmic, intense, lusty crying that is robust, vigorous, and strong in sound.

AA: Should the infant move into a prolonged respiratory pause, e.g., beyond 8 seconds, AA should be marked. The infant has removed him or herself from the state continuum.

More than one box per 2-minute time block can be marked, depending on the fluctuation and behavior the infant shows. Operationally, typically a 2-second to 3-second duration of a behavioral configuration is necessary to be registered as a distinct state; however, even briefer excursions, especially into states 4 and 6, can be recorded reliably.

Attention-Related Behaviors

These behaviors are often either related to attentional states and seem to be signs of still poor modulation, such as fussing, sneezing, yawning, or they are the expression of various levels of attentional availability, such as eye floating, ooh face, etc.

Fuss: While fussing is often a component of state 5 behavior, this is not necessarily so. At times fussing occurs in state 3 or even in state 2. fussing is an audible vocal expression of discomfort, uneasiness, unhappiness, and/or upset.

Yawn: The infant opens the mouth widely, usually with a deep inspiration.

Sneeze: The infant expels air forcibly from the mouth and nose in an explosive, spasmodic, involuntary action.

Face open: The infant either with eyes open or eyes closed lifts the eyebrows high up. This may occur in sleep state or in awake state.

Eye Floating: The infant's eyes move in floating, apparently involuntary fashion, often disjugately. This may be in semi-open eye position or with fully open eyes.

Avert: The infant actively averts the eyes from a social target. The infant may momentarily close them.

Frown: The infant knits the eyebrows or darkens the eyes by contracting the periocular musculature, engaging in a flexion of the upper face.

Ooh Face: The infant rounds the mouth and purses the lips or extends them in an ooh configuration. This may be with eyes opened or closed.

Locking: The infant locks onto an object or sight in the environment or his caregiver, or may be maintaining a steady gaze fastened in one direction. The sound component of an environmental event may appear to contribute to the locking.

Cooing: The infant emits a soft, pleasurable, modulated cooing sound.

Speech Movements: The infant's tongue and lips move in soft, rhythmical, speech-like fashion, while the face is typically relaxed and animated, or the gaze is animatedly engaged with the environment.

3

A CONCEPTUAL FRAMEWORK FOR INTERVENTIONS WITH LOW BIRTHWEIGHT PREMATURE CHILDREN AND THEIR FAMILIES

CRAIG T. RAMEY
DARLENE L. SHEARER

Approximately 200,000 preterm infants are born annually in the United States. About 6% of all live births in the white and 12% in the nonwhite population are considered low birthweight (LBW), that is, weighing 2,500 g or less. About 1% of white and 2%–3% of nonwhite infants weigh 1,500 g or less and are considered very low birthweight or VLBW (McCormick, 1985). The incidence of prematurity and LBW has remained surprisingly unchanged over the past 25 years. Reductions in neonatal mortality, however, are steadily increasing the prevalence of biologically vulnerable infants in the overall population (Bennett, 1988). Today's neonatal intensive care units (NICUs) are "becoming increasingly populated by tiny newborns [< 1,000 g] who breathe spontaneously, oxygenate effectively, and are likely to survive well beyond the neonatal period. . . . These are medically stable yet extremely fragile infants whose central nervous systems . . . are immature and vulnerable." (Gilkerson, Gorski, & Panitz, 1990, p. 1470).

Current data continue to indicate that preterm and VLBW infants are at increased risk for a multiplicity of problems, such as prolonged stays in NICUs (Gorski, 1991), rehospitalization in the first year of life (Kitchen et al., 1990), delayed or abnormal development (Escobar, Littenberg, & Petitti, 1991; Infant Health and Development Project [IHDP], 1990), and minor neurodevelopmental and neurobehavioral sequelae, now referred to as the "new morbidity" of prematurity (Bennett, 1988, p. 223).

For many years the immediate major challenges to care of preterm infants concerned resuscitation and survival. During the past decade as the number of surviving infants with lower gestational age has increased, the prevention of biomedical and psychological problems associated with increased prematurity has received growing research attention, including the provision of developmental interventions in the NICU and after discharge. Indeed, some experts suggest these infants require developmental care equal to their acute and chronic medical care (Dudley et al., 1993; Gilkerson et al., 1990). The rationale for specific early interventions is frequently complicated and highly technical. However, the general ideas behind many of these interventions have much in common. This chapter provides a broad conceptual framework for better understanding of developmental and familial interventions to enhance the immediate and long-term outcomes during the first three years of life.

IDENTIFICATION OF THE AT-RISK AND VULNERABLE PRETERM INFANT

Systematic intervention is a necessary step in the treatment of prematurity. Since the 1950s, as a result of greater understanding of perinatal pathophysiology, many therapeutic interventions used in treating premature infants have been developed. Neonatology has evolved through the rapid proliferation of astonishing technical advances that allow even the tiniest infants to survive. Systematic intervention, including developmental intervention, is a significant alteration of ongoing life processes. Painful and costly errors such as those that led to the discovery of retrolental fibroplasia and bronchopulmonary dysplasia serve to remind us that even apparently appropriate caretaking practices in the nursery may lead to developmental disaster (Cone, 1985). For this reason, a major concern of the developmental interventionist is the accurate identification of those infants who will require developmental or familial interventions to achieve optimal development and the simultaneous minimization of iatrogenic effects.

Infants who require such interventions are referred to as "at-risk" or "high-risk" infants. Used in this context, these terms refer to infants who are at risk for developmental delay or disability as a result of factors occurring during pregnancy, at birth, or in the postnatal period. "At risk" does not describe the specific developmental disorder or developmental pathway. The term does not indicate the type of severity of developmental problems for which the infant is at risk. Nor does it imply necessarily that the infant will experience developmental problems. In most cases at risk serves as a probabilistic indicator of the potential for developmental vulnerability (Meisels & Wasik, 1990).

Although numerous older studies indicate the premature or LBW infant is at high risk for adverse developmental sequelae (Caputo & Mandell, 1970; Cornell & Gottfried, 1976; Knobloch & Pasamanick, 1966; Weiner, 1966), the cognitive developmental outcome may not necessarily be below-average performance even without developmental or familial interventions (Francis-Williams & Davis, 1962; Phillips, 1972; Rabinovitch, Bibace, & Chaplan, 1961). Even the VLBW infant may, in fact, meld successfully into the general population (Taub, Caputo, & Goldstein, 1975) and be able to attend regular schools (Kitchen, et al., 1980; Klein, et al., 1985; Lefebvre et al., 1988; Saigal et al., 1991). This melding is particularly likely if premature and LBW infants are born into knowledgeable and economically and socially resourceful families (Brooks-Gunn et al., 1993; IHDP, 1990).

The question of where risk principally lies is a source of debate. On the one hand, severity of medical illness in the postnatal period appears important for preterm infants (IHDP, 1990; Paneth et al. 1982; Siegel, 1982), as does gestational age and LBW in view of the greater number of medical interventions performed and the subsequent morbidity in this group (Dudley et al., 1993). On the other hand, problems during pregnancy and labor are not *necessarily* associated with childhood physical and psychological disorders, as was believed 25 years ago. The concept of a continuum of "reproductive casualty" (Pasamanick & Knobloch, 1961) has been complemented by one of "caretaking casualty" (Sameroff & Chandler, 1975), in which the problems and positive contributions of the postnatal environment are also weighed in predicting long-term outcomes for children.

Are all preterm and LBW infants appropriate targets for developmental intervention, and, if not, what criteria are to be used by those who provide intervention? Given what is currently known about the contributions of biological/biomedical risk factors and that of sociological/psychological risk factors, these questions cannot be answered in a simple, straightforward manner.

In identifying infants at high risk, one must recognize that the attributes or characteristics of preterm infants are not necessarily constant across cohorts or within cohorts over time. For example, surviving VLBW infants (i.e., less than 1,500 grams) did not exist in quantity 25 years ago, as they do routinely now. As more information is discovered about their long-term developmental adaptation through longitudinal follow-up, we are learning that while some of these children experience major neuromotor abnormalities, which are seemingly proportionate or result from the degree of biological insult, many others experience a wide range of learning and behavior problems that are not fully attributable to the degree of apparent insult (Klein, Hack, & Breslau, 1989). Prematurity cannot be described as a singular concept, or as a specific syndrome with well-defined characteristics and developmental sequelae. Because of this critical factor, one cannot necessarily compute a higher level of risk contingent solely on a greater degree of prematurity. Furthermore, with improved medical care, the characteristics and abilities of small preterm infants have changed significantly. Technological advances in care such as the use of high-frequency ventilators and exogenous administration of natural or synthetic surfactant have resulted in tiny, spontaneously breathing and oxygenating infants whose physiologic immaturity of all other organ systems makes them highly vulnerable for a longer period of time.

Changes in the NICU environment itself have increased the numbers and characteristics of VLBW infants who survive. Many neonatal nurseries have made concerted efforts to modify their physical environment with particular attention to noise pollution, ambient light exposure, organization of care and handling, and diurnal rhythms. Thus, differential survival rates across cohorts may affect the modal attributes of populations from which samples are drawn. Similarly, as development progresses within a cohort over time, characteristics of the preterm infant may change relative to the term infant. Preterm infants may show markedly deficient performance at an early point in development, yet show average or above-average performance (relative to their peers) at later ages and vice versa. Thus, risk is not likely constant throughout development or across cohorts, particularly in a changing environment of therapeutic practice. Also, LBW and premature infants are more likely to occur in some cultural and subpopulation groups than others, and this increased incidence may have predictable associations with the likelihood of poverty and other changing factors (Klerman, in press).

The important points to be made from these observations, points that will be emphasized throughout this chapter, concern the concept of high risk. First, the concept of high risk is a probabilistic one based on currently known outcomes. Second, the probability of the development of a specific condition may change as medical practices and environmental quality change during development and across cohorts and population subgroups. Thus, a conceptualization of the attributes of a given population as it exists now is important if one is to understand which interventions may be appropriate. Third, the attributes of the individual infant develop and change over developmental time. Interventions must therefore be based on frequent and repeated observations, flexibility to meet changing circumstances, and constant attention to possible side effects (Landesman and Ramey, 1989). For these reasons, identification of infants' biomedical and behavioral attributes and the causal mechanisms by which they develop is a necessary step to appropriate and needed developmental intervention strategies designed to reduce morbidity associated with prematurity and LBW.

Because so many factors potentially affect the growth and development of preterm infants, we have found it helpful to develop a general model to make more explicit our approach to the factors that potentially regulate development in the neonatal and postneonatal period. We propose this model as an aid to understanding the development of preterm infants and how developmental interventions in the NICU, and later, might enhance it. We call this model, based on our earlier work in developmental systems theory as applied to LBW and premature infants (Ramey et al 1984a, 1985b; Ramey, Zeskind, & Hunter, 1982) a Biosocial Developmental Systems Framework, presented schematically in Figure 3.1.

DESCRIPTION OF THE MODEL

It is important to note that we construe this general model as evolving itself. The model has two main functions: first, to provide a device with which one can summarize the current state of knowledge concerning factors that promote or retard biologic, social, and cognitive development in infants during the prenatal and subsequent postnatal period; second, to serve as a guide for the selection of research topics to increase that body of knowledge.

Within this developmental systems approach, we are concerned with five levels of variables across the neonatal period and beyond: (1) the genetic, prenatal, medical, sociocultural, and community histories of the infant (and parent); (2) the prolonged hospitalization or exposure to a variety of medical, developmental,

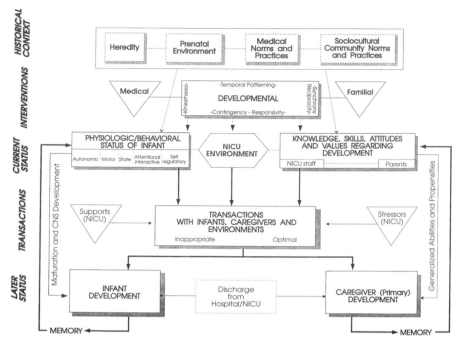

Figure 3.1. Biosocial developmental systems framework for low birth-weight/premature infants.

and familial interventions; (3) the current status of developmental expectations and behavioral propensities of caregivers at any given time as well as the current status of the infant; (4) behavioral transactions among the infant and significant others within the context of the NICU environment; and (5) future status of the child and his or her primary caregivers in the context of the home environment.

Multiple influences from conception onward are recognized as important in this model. We hypothesize, however, that the behavioral interactions between infants and adults are the most important normative influence on cognitive and social development. This development, guided primarily by the infant/caregiver interactions, typically occurs throughout infancy and early childhood until a child acquires the cognitive sophistication to regulate his or her own development through activities such as engaging in conversation or acquiring reading proficiency. For the preterm infant and the array of caregivers in the NICU, these interactions are substantially different in terms of their specific properties, time of onset, and frequency. The characteristics of each of the contributors to this transactional process—infant, caregiver (parent or professional), and environment—interact in multiple and complex ways to produce the transaction, which may range from inappropriate to optimal, depending on the fit of each contributor. The manner in which they interact and the role of intervention in enhancing the transaction will be discussed in the next section. It is important to note that family and environmental stresses and supports impinge on infant/caregiver transactions in ways that enhance or limit the child's potential development. Based on this conceptualization, the caregiver-child-environment interaction prevails as the key influence on how well a child achieves maximum developmental potential.

Caregivers bring to potential behavioral transactions many expectations and behavioral propensities, both general and child-specific, that potentially influence infant-caregiver transactions. In the NICU setting, examples of behavioral propensities might include staff characteristics, such as employment experience, personal flexibility, or cultural competence in working with families whose values and lifestyle may differ from their own, and parent factors, such as physical discomfort, personal coping patterns, preparedness for parenting, and individual need. As another example, mothers' educational levels and cognitive abilities as general propensities have been related to the cognitive outcomes of LBW infants (Ramey & Ramey, 1992). Similarly, a parent's use of developmental encouragement and specific knowledge of altered response cues and developmental milestones of preterm infants may positively affect the cognitive outcome of a LBW infant (Brazelton, 1986). This may occur, in part, because such parents would potentially have a broader behavioral repertoire themselves for fostering good state organization in the infants for whom they care, thus promoting better transactions with the infant (Horowitz, 1990). The infant, with good state organization, could benefit in his transactions with his environment.

Developmental and familial interventions may directly or indirectly modify one or more of the characteristics of infants and their caregivers. Knowing that LBW infants are rated as less socially responsive than normal birthweight babies and that mothers of preterm infants tend to display less positive affect, a systematic intervention might improve transactions by changing both parents' expectations and behaviors. Any intervention perceived by a mother as increased social support might also positively affect the LBW infant by altering her behavior toward the infant.

Figure 3.2 provides an application of the Biosocial Developmental Systems Framework to interventions for premature and LBW infants and their families. This more specific model is intended to illustrate several points. First, biological and social risk factors have different relationships to adverse outcomes during development. Throughout the period of early prenatal development, biologic risk factors such as chromosomal damage, infections, and other biological events are more likely to be associated with poor outcomes, whereas social risk factors such as parental education, economic factors, and specific behavior patterns (with the exception of drug use) more likely take a developmental toll later in a child's development. Over time both biological and social risk factors generally gravitate toward moderate or low levels of risk. Variations in the stabilized risk levels of biologic and social factors for subpopulations depend in large part on cultural and institutional contexts such as availability of nutrition, medical care, schooling, family support services, violent crime, and so forth.

Within this biosocial risk context we consider three interventions traditionally provided in the NICU (e.g., medical, developmental, and familial) and attempt

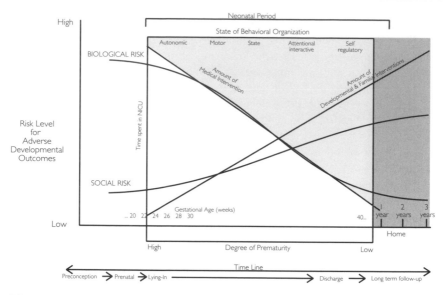

Figure 3.2. Conceptual relationship of NICU interventions and risk for adverse development outcomes.

to show their relationship to factors such as the degree of prematurity, stage of behavioral organization, amount of time spent in the NICU environment, and the contrast of these factors with the amount of time spent in the home environment. These interventions are likely introduced at different points in development and to have, normatively speaking, different average durations depending, in part, on the likely initial state or characteristics of the infant and family, the severity of the adverse developmental outcome, and availability of resources. The three forms of intervention may overlap in application, and we separate them here for conceptual clarity. They are (1) medical interventions (2) developmental interventions and (3) familial interventions. What remains unanswered in this model is the relationship of events (including the naturally occuring risk indicators and the interventions used to address them) that occur during the time the infant spends in the NICU and the developmental outcomes identified long after hospital discharge through neonatal follow-up. Are they related, and, if so, what are the causal mechanisms? It has been assumed that developmental outcomes observed at three years of age are directly associated with events in an infant's early neonatal period, when biological risk is at its highest point. However, with the current evidence and emphasis of ecological influences on development, it might be better for the practitioner to consider experiences the infant likely encounters in the home environment during the critical developmental years of early childhood. The degree and intensity of interventions planned with this approach need to take social risk into account at least as fully as the initial biological risk. This proportion is obviously addressable through systematic, longitudinal empirical studies.

IMPLICATIONS OF THE BIOSOCIAL SYSTEMS MODEL FOR MEDICAL, DEVELOPMENT, AND FAMILIAL INTERVENTIONS

Medical Interventions

Although the rapid proliferation and sophistication of technical advances have greatly enhanced the scientific basis of medical care of the high-risk neonate over the past 30 years (Hack et al., 1983), the guiding principles for medical interventions of neonates have remained the same: survival and simultaneous minimization of damage.

Follow-up studies reported mainly in the 1990s have forced us to face new issues in medical interventions, such as the quality of life for NICU survivors. Medical technology solved the immediate problems of survival faced, for example, by 23-and 24-week-old fetuses. Intensive and specialized care has also meant that infants are being subjected to increasingly more intrusive and vigorous investigations and treatments (Wolke, 1987) and may remain in the NICU environment for many months. As we have redefined the accepted limits of viability, we have also created a population of infants at increasing risk for retinopathy of prematurity, short gut syndrome, hydrocephalus, to name a few, and whose ultimate developmental and intellectual status is cause for serious concern. We are still trying to learn if delicate organ systems are altered because an important part of the development occurs in an isolette instead of the womb (Gorski, 1991).

With each decade of advances in medical interventions, we find that LBW infants present a case in which intervention helps an immature organism to adapt to an environment for which it may be unprepared. By virtue of its anachronous birth, the premature infant is thrust into a position that has no *naturally occurring* support system. The knowledge and response of professionals in providing artificial support must be fabricated and, by definition, proceed by approximations based on trial and error. Empiricism is thus a necessity and characterizes the currently operating, inductive theoretical approach that organizes the medical approach to the care of this population. This empirical approach, with its frequent monitoring of infant attributes, may provide the basis for the approach to continued medical and other interventions once the infant leaves the nursery. Within the context of this chapter and the systems framework presented here, it seems appropriate to suggest that outcomes associated with medical interventions not be viewed in isolation from developmental and familial interventions. Medical care and treatment must avoid overloading the immature nervous system just as it supports other vital homeostatic mechanisms associated with survival.

opmental Interventions

acreased survival of smaller and more preterm infants compelled researchers to consider the impact of the nursery environment and accompanying caregiving practices on the long-term developmental status of the LBW infant. The underlying theories that dominated modifications of the environment and care have attempted to (1) normalize and humanize the disruptive effects of the NICU to resemble the environment of term newborns (e.g., Barnett et al., 1970; Beckwith et al., 1976; Field, 1977); (2) correct for presumed sensory deprivation endured by the preterm newborn in the NICU and thereby optimize subsequent development and decrease the likelihood of long-term neurodevelopmental sequelae (e.g., Katz, 1971; Kramer, et al., 1975; Leib, Benfield, & Guidubaldi, 1980; Scarr-Salapatek & Williams, 1973); and (3) compensate for intrauterine experiences lost as a result of premature birth (Korner, Kraemer, & Haffner, 1975; Korner, Guilleminault, & Van den Hoed, 1978).

Some popular views of the intensive care environment suggest that it is (1) a place of sensory deprivation and therefore requiring a variety of supplemental stimulations such as auditory, kinesthetic, tactile, visual, and vestibular (Campbell, 1983; Katz, 1971; Korner et al., 1975; Kramer & Pierpont, 1976 Neal, 1968; Rice; 1977; Segall, 1972); (2) a place of constant overstimulation and therefore suggesting less handling and less intervention of all types or at least extreme caution when providing stimulation (Als, Lawhon, & Brown, 1986; Gorski, 1982; Gorski, Leonard, & Sweet, 1984); or (3) an environment of inappropriate patterns of interactions, including examples of both deprivation and overstimulation, and therefore suggesting more attention be made to observing and interpreting response behaviors of the infant (Als et al., 1986; Huntington & Gorski, 1988; Linn, Howowitz, & Fox, 1985).

In the Biosocial Development Systems Framework that we have presented, developmental interventions—regardless of their theoretical basis—will directly affect the transactions that occur between the infant, the NICU environment, and the caregivers (professional and parent). The appropriateness of specific developmental interventions is debated throughout the following chapters in this book. We believe, however, that the effectiveness of the intervention will be potentially attenuated by the same components the intervention is designed to affect: an infant's physiological and behavioral status and neuromaturational stage, the physical environment itself, and the contributions and characteristics of the caregiver. But these are simply matters for systematic empirical inquiry.

Almost all of the studies of developmental interventions thus far have had methodological weaknesses that challenge their clinical utility and generalizability to today's NICU care (Gilkerson et al., 1990; Lacy & Ohlsson, 1993). Apart from short-term physiological and psychological effects, the emerging evidence of these studies shows that our understanding of the factors actually responsible for these changes is seriously limited. It also suggests that the methods by which we measure these effects may be inadequate in capturing the complexity of so many variables and interactions. There is still little hard evidence about how the nursery environment affects preterm infants in general (Wolke, 1987). The reviewed evidence does suggest a bad fit between the NICU environment and an infant's behavioral organization and implies that a more comprehensive and individualized perspective on neonatal intensive care, putting procedures in a developmentally appropriate framework of care, is paramount. In spite of these constraints, the NICU should be viewed as a critical site for early intervention to optimize an infant's development and a family's adaptation to an unexpected, complicated, and stressful event—the arrival of a LBW premature, acutely ill child.

Familial Interventions

Historically speaking, nurseries caring for preterm infants have been preoccupied with meeting the physical rather than social and emotional needs of infants and, to a minimal or nonexistent degree, the needs of parents. Earlier considerations of parents frequently neglected their role and needs in the interest of maintaining a sterile environment to promote LBW infant survival. Parents and other family members were viewed as potential sources of infection, and their presence in the nursery was, therefore, minimized by strict isolation policies. Even when these policies changed to permit formal visiting hours, parents were viewed by hospital staff as "necessary" obstacles, to be suffered and worked around. The idea that parents are critical, within the context of the NICU, to an infant's survival did not evolve until recently.

A much publicized book by Marshall Klaus and John Kennell (1976) proposed that a sensitive period occurred within the first minutes and hours of every infant's life that subsequently influenced the development of a bond between parent and child and the long-term outcome of their relationship. As a result of this and other studies (e.g., Goldberg, 1982; Leiderman, 1982), preterm infants were perceived as a particularly vulnerable population for attachment problems.

While early contact with their infant may enhance parents' initial experiences and facilitate early parent-infant relationships, few lasting effects have been accurately measured (Goldberg, 1982, Hunt, Cooper, & Tooley, 1988; Leiderman, 1982; Levy-Shiff, Sharir, & Mogilner, 1989). Parents, despite being allowed to visit their child in the nursery, often suffer severe emotional stress (Minde et al., 1980; Newman, 1980), and the level of their distress is usually unrelated to the staff-perceived clinical severity of their infant's problems (Benfield, Leib, & Reuter, 1976).

The critical role of parents in the continued health and development of their LBW infant beyond the neonatal period, long after hospital discharge, however, has been well documented (Beckwith et al., 1976; IHDP, 1990; Ramey et al., 1992; Rauh et al., 1988; Sameroff & Seifer, 1983). As a result, parent and parent-infant intervention programs have been implemented to indirectly influence the parent-infant interaction by targeting parental perceptions and responses (Minde et al., 1980; Zeskind & Iacino, 1984) or to directly affect interaction by providing skill training and sensitivity coaching, thereby facilitating parents' attunement to their infants (Rauh et al., 1990).

The Biosocial Developmental Systems Framework suggests that parents encumbered by limited education or intellectual capacity, poverty, poor social support, mental illness, personality disorder, or distorted or defective affective experiences in their own childhood will have considerable difficulty in conducting normal transactions with their infant. Familial interventions to support caregivers in meaningful and normative transactions are, therefore, critical to developmental outcomes of both the infant and caregiver. Such interventions, if they are to prevent developmental disasters, must begin as early in an infant's existence as possible and must be viewed as an ongoing process.

CONCLUSION

Having discussed three types of interventions that potentially affect the long-term development of LBW and preterm infants and viewed them in the context of medical and social risk, we emphasize the following points.

1. Biological and socioenvironmental risk factors interact with other parts of a larger ecosystem that make up the infant's future (Bronfenbrenner, 1989). It is critical, therefore, that the posthospital or post-NICU period be viewed as one in which behavioral transactions play a significant role, or not, in achievement of maximum developmental potential. Professionals who provide intervention and care within the NICU may fail to view the posthospital period as an important part of the LBW infant's continuum of development (Gilkerson et al., 1990). A "hierarchy of activities" (Gilkerson et al., 1990, p. 446) clearly exists in the NICU in which life-threatening situations take precedence over all other activities. Hence, activities in the postcritical phase of an infant's life, such as parent teaching, identification of an infant's and family's needs in preparation for discharge, and mobilization of community resources to facilitate the transition home, may be shortchanged, if not totally overlooked, if there is no systematic and valued provision for such planning.
2. Interactions and transactions of the infant and caregiver during the developmental period of language acquisition, cognitive learning, and self-esteem building are more critically linked to how well the child performs in school than the degree of overstimulation or understimulation encountered in the NICU. However, the first early interactions and transactions that occur between infant and caregiver take place in the NICU and likely have a lasting impact by laying the groundwork for future transactions.
3. Several major principles that have been identified as critical for effective intervention programs (Ramey and Ramey, 1992) may be applied to this discussion of developmental interventions in the NICU. These principles are based on studies of children from economically impoverished families, children with combined environmental and biological risks, and children with disabilities identified during infancy.
   The principle of timing. Generally, interventions that begin earlier and

continue longer afford greater benefits. In the NICU, timing of developmental intervention can optimize maturation by reducing exposure to destabilizing stressors and structuring the environment to support physiological, motor, and behavioral state systems.

The principle of intensity. More intensive interventions, as indexed by variables such as the number of hours per day, produce larger positive effects (in cognitive and social performance) than do less intensive interventions. Developmental care in the nursery could be viewed as an example of intensity. If it becomes a pervasive orientation of all care procedures toward maintaining the infant in as organized or stable a condition as possible and managing the physical and social environment to minimize stressors, it is likely to produce effects such as improved medical and growth outcomes, shorter hospital stay, and improved behavioral organization at discharge.

The principle of breadth. Interventions that provide more comprehensive services and use multiple routes to enhance infant development generally have stronger effects. The use of developmental care as an effective developmental intervention embraces multiple approaches such as reducing sources of environmental stress, reducing physiological and behavioral destabilization associated with behavioral handling, supporting motor development, and supporting organization of sleep/wake states. However, viewing the infant in the context of the family to which he or she belongs necessitates that effective intervention must also include other services such as health and social services, transportation, assistance with meeting urgent needs, and parent support.

The principle of individual differences. Developmental care emphasizes that all aspects of intervention are ideally provided based on cues from the infant; therefore, it is tailored to an infant's unique needs rather than as a standard recipe to specific outcomes.

The principle of environmental maintenance of development. Developmental care provided only to an infant in the NICU will, at best, likely produce short-term effects that will probably dissipate over time unless the parent understands and uses these same and more sophisticated principles later at home.

In conclusion, we emphasize that the care and treatment of the LBW and premature child is a complex and demanding interdisciplinary task. It requires informed cooperation between parents and professionals and sustained compassionate care for the developing child. Such care is both a labor of love and a mark of a truly civilized culture—one that uses science in the service of human development.

REFERENCES

Als, H., Lawhon, G., & Brown, E. (1986). Individualized behavioral and environmental care for the very low birth weight preterm infant at high risk for bronchopulmonary dysplasia: neonatal intensive care unit and developmental outcome. *Pediatrics, 78*, 1123–1132.

Barnett, C. R., Leiderman, P. H., Grobstein, R., & Klaus, M. H. (1970). Neonatal separation: the maternal side of interactional deprivation. *Pediatrics, 45*, 197–205.

Beckwith, L., Cohen, S. E., Kopp, C. B., Parmelee, A. H., & Marcy, T. (1976). Caregiver-infant interaction and early cognitive development in preterm infants. *Child Dev, 47*, 579–587.

Benfield, D. G., Leib, S. A., & Reuter J. (1976). Grief response of parents following referral of the critically ill newborn. *N Engl J Med, 294*, 975–978.

Bennett, F. C. (1988). Neurodevelopmental outcome in low birthweight infants: the role of development intervention. In R. D. Guthrie (Ed.), *Neonatal Intensive Care* (pp. 221–249). New York: Churchill Livingston.

Brazelton, T. B. (1986). Development of newborn behavior. In F. Falkner & J. M. Tanner (Eds.), *Human Growth* (Vol. 2, pp. 519–540). New York: Plenum Publishing.

Bronfenbrenner, U. (1989). Ecological systems theory. In R. Vasta (Ed.), *Annals of Child Development* (pp. 187–249). Greenwich, CT: JAI Press.

Brooks-Gunn, J., Gross, R. T., Kraemer, H. C. Spiker, D., & Shapiro, S. (1992). Enhancing the cognitive outcomes of low birth weight, premature infants: for whom is the intervention most effective? *Pediatrics, 89*, 1209–1215.

Campbell, S. K. (1983). Effects of developmental intervention in the special care nursery. *Adv Dev Behav Pediatr, 4*, 165–179.

Caputo, D. V., & Mandell, W. (1970). Consequences of low birth weight. *Dev Psychol, 3*, 363–372.

Cone, T. E. (1985). *History of the Care and Feeding of the Premature Infant.* Boston: Little, Brown.

Cornell, E. H., & Gottfried, A. W. (1976). Intervention with premature human infants. *Child Dev, 47*, 32–39.

Dudley, M., Gyler, L., Blinkhorn, S., & Barnett, B. (1993). Psychosocial interventions for very low birthweight infants: their scope and efficacy. *Aust N Z J Psychiatry, 27*, 74–84.

Escobar, G. J., Littenberg, B., & Petitti, D. B. (1991). Outcome among surviving very low birthweight infants: a meta-analysis. *Arch Dis Child, 66*, 204–211.

Field, T. M. (1977). Effects of early separation, interactive deficits, and experimental manipulations on infant-mother face-to-face interaction. *Child Dev, 48*, 763–771.

Francis-Williams, J., & Davis, P. A. (1962). Very low birth weight and later intelligence. *Dev Med Child Neurol, 16*, 709–718.

Gilkerson, L., Gorski, P., & Panitz, P. (1990). Hospital-based intervention for preterm infants and their families. In S. J. Meisels & J. P. Shonkoff (Eds.), *Handbook of Early Childhood Intervention* (pp. 445–468). New York: Cambridge University Press.

Goldberg, S. (1982). Some biological aspects of early parent-infant interaction. In S. G. Moore & C. R. Cooper (Eds.), *The Young Child: Reviews in Research.* Washington, DC: National Association for the Education of Young Children.

Gorski, P. A. (1982). Premature infant behavioral and physiological responses to caregiving interventions in an intensive care nursery. In J. D. Call, E. Galenson, & R. L. Tyson (Eds.), *Frontiers of Infant Psychiatry* (pp. 256–263). New York: Basic Books.

Gorski, P. A. (1991). Developmental intervention during neonatal hospitalization. *Pediatr Clin North Am, 38(6)*, 1469–1479.

Gorski, P., Leonard, C., & Sweet, D. (1984). Caring for immature infants: a touchy subject. In C. C. Brown (Ed.), *The Many Facets of Touch*, Johnson & Johnson Pediatric Round Table #10 (pp. 84–91). Johnson and Johnson Baby Products Company. Skillman, N.J.

Hack, M., Caron, B., Rivers, A., & Fanaroff, A. A. (1983). The very low birth weight infant: the broader spectrum of morbidity during infancy and early childhood. *J Dev Behav Pediatr, 4*(4), 243–249.

Horowitz, F. D. (1990). Targeting infant stimulation efforts: theoretical challenges for research and intervention. *Clin Perinatol, 17(1),* 185–195.

Hunt, J., Cooper, B., & Tooley, W. (1988). Very low birth weight infants at 8 and 11 years of age: role of neonatal illness and family status. *Pediatrics, 82,* 596–603.

Huntington, L., & Gorski, P. A. (1988). Temporal relations between preterm infant behaviors and physiological distress. *Pediatr Res, 23,* 210a.

Infant Health and Development Program. (1990). Enhancing the outcomes of low birth weight, premature infants: a multisite randomized trial. *JAMA, 263,* 3035–3042.

Katz, V. (1971). Auditory stimulation and developmental behavior of the premature infant. *Nurs Res, 20,* 196–201.

Kitchen, W. H., Ford, G. H., Doyle, L. W., Richards, A. L., & Kelly, E. A. (1990). Health and hospital readmissions of very low birth weight and normal birth weight children. *Am J Dis Child, 144,* 213–218.

Kitchen, W. H., Ryan, M. M., Rickards, A., McDougall, A. B., Billson, F. A., Keir, E. H., & Naylor, F. D. (1980). A longitudinal study of very low-birthweight infants: an overview of performance at eight years. *Dev Med Child Neurol, 22,* 172–188.

Klaus, M. H., & Kennell, J. H. (1976). *Maternal-Infant Bonding.* Saint Louis: C. V. Mosby.

Klein, N., Hack, M., & Breslau, N. (1989). Children who were very low birth weight: development and academic achievement at nine years of age. *J Dev Behav Pediatr, 10(1),* 32–37.

Klein, N., Hack, M., Gallagher, J., & Fanaroff, A. A. (1985). Preschool performance of children with normal intelligence who were very low-birth-weight infants. *Pediatrics, 75,* 531–537.

Klerman, L. V. (1994). The impact of economic status on the health of women and children. In H. M. Wallace, R. Nelson, & P. J. Sweeney (Eds.), *Maternal and Child Health Practices* (4th ed.). Third Party Publishing: Oakland, CA.

Knobloch, H., & Pasamanick, B. (1966). Prospective studies on the epidemiology of reproductive casualty: methods, findings, and some implications. *Merrill-Palmer Q, 12,* 27–36.

Korner, A., Guilleminault, C., & Van den Hoed, J. (1978). Reduction of sleep apnea and bradycardia in preterm infants on oscillating water beds: a controlled polygraphic study. *Pediatrics, 61,* 528–533.

Korner, A., Kraemer, H., & Haffner, E. (1975). Effects of waterbed flotation on premature infants: a pilot study. *Pediatrics, 56,* 361–365.

Kramer, L. I., & Pierpont, M. E. (1976). Rocking waterbeds and auditory stimuli to enhance growth of preterm infants. *J Pediatr, 88,* 297–299.

Kramer, M., Chamorro, I., Green, D., & Knudtson, F. (1975). Extra tactile stimulation on the preterm infant. *Nursing Res, 24,* 324–334.

Lacy, J. B., & Ohlsson, A. (1993). Behavioral outcomes of environmental or care-giving hospital-based interventions for preterm infants: a critical review. *Acta Paediatr, 82,* 408–415.

Landesman, S., & Ramey, C. T. (1989). Developmental psychology and mental retardation: integrating scientific principles with treatment practices. *Am Psychol, 44,* 409–415.

Lefebvre, F., Bard, H., Veilleux, A., & Martel, C. (1988). Outcome at school age of children with birthweights of 1000 grams or less. *Dev Med Child Neurol, 30*, 170–180.

Leib, S., Benfield, G., & Guidubaldi, J. (1980). Effects of early intervention and stimulation on the preterm infant. *Pediatrics, 66*, 83–89.

Leiderman, P. H. (1982). The critical period hypothesis revisited: mother to infant social bonding in the neonatal period. In K. Immelman, G. Barlow, M. Main, & L. Petrinovich (Eds.), *Issues in Behavioral Development*. Cambridge: Cambridge University Press.

Levy-Shiff, R., Sharir, H., & Mogilner, M. B. (1989). Mother-and father-preterm infant relationship in the hospital preterm nursery. *Child Dev, 60*, 93–102.

Linn, P., Horowitz, F., & Fox, H. (1985). Stimulation in the NICU: is more necessarily better? *Clin Perinatol, 12*, 407–422.

Maisels, M. J. (1993). Foreword. In M. H. Klaus & A. A. Fanaroff (Eds.), *Care of the High-Risk Neonate* (4th ed). Philadelphia: W. B. Saunders.

McCormick, M. C. (1985). The contribution of low birth weight to infant mortality and childhood morbidity. *N Engl J Med, 312*, 82–90.

Meisels, S. J., & Wasik, B. A. (1990). Who should be served? Identifying children in need of early intervention. In S. J. Meisels & J. P. Shonkoff (Eds.), *Handbook of Early Childhood Intervention* (pp. 05–632). New York: Cambridge University Press.

Minde, K., Morton, P., Manning, D., & Hines, B. (1980). Some determinants of mother-infant interaction in the premature nursery. *J Am Acad Child Adolesc Psychiatry, 19*, 1–21.

Neal, M. (1968). Vestibular stimulation and developmental behavior of the small premature infant. *Nurs Res Report, 3*, 1–5.

Newman, L. F. (1980). Parents' perceptions of their low birth weight infants. *Paediatrician, 9*, 182–190.

Paneth, N., Kiely, J. L., Wallenstein, S., Marcus, M., Pakter, J., & Susser, M. (1982). Neonatal intensive care and neonatal mortality in low birthweight infants. *N Engl J Med, 307*, 149–155.

Pasamanick, B., & Knobloch, M. (1961). Epidemiologic studies on the complications of pregnancy and the birth process. In G. Caplan (Ed.), *Prevention of Mental Disorders in Children*. New York: Basic Books.

Phillips, M. B. (1972). Prediction of scholastic performance from perinatal and infant development indices. *Dissert Abs Int, 33*, 1526. (University Microfilms No. 72–25, 648).

Rabinovitch, M. S., Bibace, R., & Chaplan, H. (1961). Sequelae of prematurity: psychological test findings. *Can Med Assoc J, 84*, 822–824.

Ramey, C. T., Bryant, D. M., Sparling, J. J., & Wasik, B. H. (1984). A biosocial systems perspective on environmental interventions for low birth weight infants. *Clin Obstet Gynecol, 27(3)*, 672–692.

Ramey, C. T., Bryant, D. M., Sparling, J. J., & Wasik, B. H. (1985). Project CARE: a comparison of two early intervention strategies. *Top Early Child Spec Educ, 5*, 12–25.

Ramey, C. T., Bryant, D. M., Wasik, B. H., Sparling, J. J., Fendt, K. H., & LaVange, L. M. (1992). Infant health and development program for low birth weight, premature infants: program elements, family participation, and child intelligence. *Pediatrics, 3*, 454–465.

Ramey, C. T., Zeskind, P. S., & Hunter, R. (1981). Biomedical and psychosocial interventions for preterm infants. In S. I. Friedman & M. Sigman (Eds.), *Preterm Birth and Psychological Development* (pp. 395–415). New York: Academic Press.

Ramey, C. T., & Ramey, S. L. (1992). Effective early intervention. *Mental Retardation, 30*, 337–345.

Ramey, S. L., & Ramey, C. T. (1992). Early educational intervention with disadvantaged children—to what effect? *Appl Prev Psychol, 1*, 130–140.

Rauh, V. A., Achenbach, T. M., Nurcombe, B., Howell, C. T., & Teti, D. M. (1988). Minimizing adverse effects of low birthweight: four year results of an early intervention program. *Child Dev, 88*, 544–553.

Rauh, V. A., Nurcombe, B., Achenbach, T., & Howell, C. (1990). The mother-infant transaction program: the content and implications of an intervention for the mothers of low-birthweight infants. *Clin Perinatol, 17(1)*, 31–45.

Rice, D. (1977). Neurophysiological development in premature infants following stimulation. *Dev Psychol, 13*, 69–76.

Saigal, S., Szatmari, P., Rosenbaum, P., Campbell, D., & King, S. (1991). Cognitive abilities and school performance of extremely low birth weight children and matched term control children at age 8 years: a regional study. *J Pediatr, 118*, 751–760.

Sameroff, A., & Chandler, M. (1975). Reproductive risk and the continuum of caretaking casualty. In F. D. Horowitz, E. M. Hetherington, S. Scarr-Salapatek, & G. Siegel (Eds.), *Review of Child Development Research* (Vol. 4, pp. 187–243). Chicago: University of Chicago Press.

Sameroff, A. J., & Seifer, R. (1983). Familial risk and child competence. *Child Dev, 54*, 1254–1268.

Scarr-Salapatek, S., & Williams, M. (1973). The effects of early stimulation on low-birth weight infants. *Child Dev, 44*, 94–101.

Segall, M. E. (1972). Cardiac responsivity to auditory stimulation in premature infants. *Nurs Res, 21*, 15–19.

Siegel, L. (1982). Reproductive, perinatal, and environmental variables as predictors of development of preterm and full term children at 5 years. *Semin Perinatol, 6*, 274–279.

Taub, H. B., Caputo, D. V., & Goldstein, K. M. (1975). Toward a modification of the indices of neonatal prematurity. *Percept Mot Skills, 40*, 43–48.

Weiner, G. (1962). Psychologic correlates of premature birth: a review. *J Nerv Ment Dis, 134*, 129–144.

Wolke, D. (1987). Environmental and developmental neonatology. *J Reprod Infant Psychol, 5*, 17–42.

Zeskind, P., & Iacino, R. (1984). Effects of maternal visitation to preterm infants in the neonatal intensive care unit. *Child Dev, 55*, 1887–1893.

4

INFANT MASSAGE THERAPY

TIFFANY FIELD

The Calcutta mother lays her infant on his stomach on her outstretched legs and stretches his body parts individually. She applies warm water and soap to the child's legs, and then moves her hands to the arms, back, abdomen, neck, and face. The massage appears rigorous (almost rough), so it is not surprising that the infant (following swaddling) then sleeps for a long period.

The Indian infant massage is a daily routine that begins in the first days of life. Some have related the precocious motor development of these infants to their daily massage. Infant massage therapists are not surprised, for they maintain that the massage provides both stimulation and relaxation. It stimulates respiration, circulation, digestion, and elimination. They claim that massaged infants sleep more soundly and that the massage relieves gas and colic and helps the healing process during illness by easing congestion and pain.

Infant massage is a common child care practice in many parts of the world, especially Asia and Africa. For example, infants are massaged for several months in Nigeria, Uganda, India, Bali, Fiji, New Guinea, New Zealand (the Maiori), Venezuela, and the Soviet Union (Auckett, 1981). In most of these countries the infant is given a massage with oil following the daily bath and prior to sleep time.

In the Western world (in Eurocentric cultures?) infant massage has only recently been discovered and researched. In the United States, for example, massage therapy schools are beginning to teach infant massage. Infant massage therapists have founded a national organization of approximately 4,000 therapists, who in turn are setting up institutes to teach parents infant massage. The techniques they use are based primarily on the teachings of two massage thera pists who trained in India (Amelia Auckett, who published a book on infant massage in 1981, and Vimala Schneider McClure, who published a similar book in 1989).

Although these infant massage training groups are located now in most regions of the United States, very little research has been conducted on the use of infant massage with healthy infants. Nonetheless, Auckett (1981) and McClure (1989) have anecdotally reported that massage (1) facilitates the parent-infant bonding process in the development of warm, positive relationships; (2) reduces stress responses to painful procedures such as inoculations; (3) reduces pain associated with teething and constipation; (4) reduces colic; (5) helps induce sleep; and (6) makes parents "feel good" while they are massaging their infants. They also report that infants who are blind or deaf become more aware of their bodies and that infants born prematurely and infants with cerebral palsy also benefit by more organized motor activity.

MASSAGE THERAPY RESEARCH WITH HIGH-RISK INFANTS

In the following sections, research findings are presented on massage therapy with preterm infants, neonates exposed to cocaine and HIV, and infants who have been abused or neglected. Data are also presented on the positive effects for the person who gives the massage and on the infant-adult relationship.

Massage Therapy with Preterm Infants

Most of the data on the positive effects of infant massage come from studies on preterm infants. During the last two decades, a number of investigators have researched the effects of massage therapy (earlier called tactile/kinesthetic stimulation) on the preterm newborn (Barnard & Bee, 1983; Rausch, 1981; Rice, 1977; Solkoff & Matuszuk, 1975; White & LaBarba, 1976). Generally, the results published by these investigators have been positive. A recent meta-analysis on 19 of these stimulation studies (Ottenbacher et al., 1987) estimated that 72% of infants receiving some form of tactile stimulation were positively affected. Most of these investigators reported greater weight gain and better performance on developmental tasks for the preterm infants receiving massage therapy. Interestingly, those who did not report significant weight gain used a light stroking procedure, which we have since found is aversive to babies, probably because it is experienced as a tickle stimulus. Investigators who reported weight gain were providing more pressure, probably stimulating both tactile and pressure receptors.

One of the studies used in this meta-analysis was conducted in our laboratory starting in 1984. In that study 40 preterm growing neonates were given 45 minutes of massage per day (in three 15-minute periods) for 10 days (Field et al., 1986). The infants averaged 31 weeks gestational age, 1,280 birth weight, and 20 days of neonatal intensive care prior to the time of the study. They were recruited for the study when they had graduated from the "Grower Nursery" at a time when their primary agenda was to gain weight. The massage sessions included three 5-minute phases. During the first and third phases, tactile stimulation was given. The newborn was placed in a prone position and given moderate pressure stroking of the head and face region, neck and shoulders, back, legs, and arms for five 1-minute segments. The Swedish-like massage was given because, as already noted, infants preferred some degree of pressure, probably because light stroking is experienced as a tickle stimulus. The middle phase

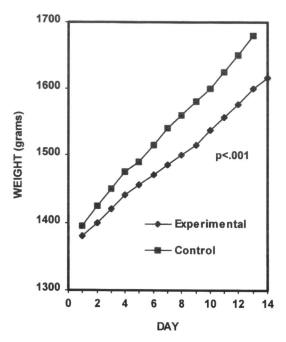

Figure 4.1 Mean daily weight of control and experimental groups to show weight gain associated with infant massage.

(kinesthetic phase) involved flexing of the infant's limbs (moving them into flexion and then extension much like bicycling motions) while the infant was lying on his or her back.

The results of this study (see Figure 4.1 taken from Field et al., 1986) suggested that the massaged infants gained 47% more weight even though the groups did not differ in calorie intake. The massaged infants were awake and active a greater percentage of the observation time, much to our surprise, because we had expected that massage would induce a soporific state leading to increased sleep time, reduced energy expenditure, and a consequent weight gain. The massaged infants showed better performance on the Brazelton scale on habituation, orientation, motor activity, and regulation of state behavior. The massaged infants, moreover, were hospitalized six days less than the control infants, yielding a hospital cost savings of approximately $3,000 per infant.

Massaging Cocaine-Exposed Preterm Infants

In the interim, a relative newcomer to the neonatal intensive care unit (NICU), the cocaine-exposed preterm infant, represent another group of infants who could presumably be helped by massage therapy. In this study the same type of massage was administered three times daily for a 10-day period with the hope that much the same effects would occur. The data suggested the following (see

Table 4.1. Means and Standard Deviations for the Brazelton Clusters and Performance

	Massage				Control			
	Day 1		Day 10		Day 1		Day 10	
	Means	SD	Means	SD	Means	SD	Means	SD
Habituation	5.7	1.2	6.0	1.0	6.6	0.5	6.4	0.8
Orientation	3.9	2.2	4.9	1.5	3.2	2.5	3.2	2.4
Motor maturity	3.8	1.0	5.0	0.6	3.7	2.0	3.4	0.9
Range of state	3.6	1.1	4.1	0.9	2.7	1.2	3.5	1.1
Regulation of state	4.6	1.6	6.9	1.0	3.0	1.2	4.8	1.2
Autonomic	5.8	1.2	5.7	1.8	5.2	2.8	5.4	1.1
Relfexes*	2.9	1.9	1.5	1.5	2.6	1.2	4.4	3.5
Stress behaviors**	2.7	1.0	1.6	0.7	2.2	1.0	2.3	1.0

*Significance for interaction effects.
**Lower score optimal.

Table 4.1 taken from Wheeden et al., 1993): (1) the massaged versus the control group cocaine-exposed preterm infants had fewer postnatal complications and exhibited fewer stress behaviors during the 10-day period; (2) they had a 28% greater daily weight gain; and (3) they demonstrated more mature motor behavior on the Brazelton exam at the end of the 10-day period (Wheeden et al., 1993).

Massaging HIV-Exposed Neonates

More recent newcomers to the NICU are HIV-exposed infants. Dr. Scafidi and our colleagues investigated whether massage therapy given by parents could improve the mental, motor, and social development of these infants. Furthermore, they investigated whether massage gave the mothers a sense of worth and reduced guilt feelings for having transmitted this disease to their infants (Scafidi & Field, 1995). We noted very impressive compliance on the part of the HIV mothers, almost 100% compliance in their administering three massages per day to their infants for the first two weeks of life. The data suggest the following (see Table 4.2): (1) greater weight gain for the massaged infants; (2) better performance on the habituation motor range of state and autonomic stability clusters of the Brazelton scale; and (3) better performance on the stress behavior scale, including alert responsiveness, cost of attention, examiner persistence, state regulation, motor tone, and excitability.

LOOKING FOR UNDERLYING MECHANISMS

Understanding the underlying mechanism for the massage therapy/weight gain relationship is critical for more widespread adoption of the therapy. Our collaborator Saul Schanberg has been conducting studies with Cynthia Kuhn at Duke

Table 4.2. Means for Brazelton Neonatal Behavior Assessment Scale
Scores and Daily Weight Gain

	Massage		Control		
Brazelton Score	*Day 1*	*Day 10*	*Day 1*	*Day 10*	p
Habituation	6.9$_a$	6.8$_a$	6.2$_a$	4.6$_b$	.01
Orientation	3.6$_a$	4.5$_a$	3.8$_a$	4.4$_a$	NS
Motor	4.3$_a$	5.2$_b$	3.8$_a$	4.5$_a$	.001
Range of state	3.5$_a$	4.3$_b$	3.2$_a$	3.6$_a$	.05
Regulation of state	4.7$_a$	4.0$_a$	5.4$_a$	4.5$_a$	NS
Autonomic stability	5.8$_a$	6.2$_b$	6.0$_a$	5.0$_a$	.003
Reflexes*	3.3$_a$	2.2$_a$	3.2$_a$	2.7$_a$	NS
Stress behaviors*	2.4$_a$	1.8$_b$	1.8$_b$	3.6$_a$	.004
Excitability*	2.5$_a$	1.5$_b$	1.8$_b$	3.2$_a$	.01
Depression*	3.5$_a$	3.0$_a$	4.8$_a$	2.9$_a$	NS
Daily weight gain	22.5$_a$	33.4$_b$	20.2$_a$	26.3$_a$	.01

*Lower score is optimal.
**Subscripts indicate significant differences between columns.

University on an animal model, removing rat pups from their mother to investigate touch deprivation and attempting to simulate the mother's behavior to restore the physiology and biochemistry of the rat pups to normal. In several studies, they noted a decrease in growth hormone (Schanberg & Field, 1988). This decrease was noted in all body organs including heart, liver, and brain (including cerebrum, cerebellum, and brain stem), and these values returned to normal once the pups were stimulated. A graduate student/animal caretaker observed rat mothers' nocturnal behavior and noted that they frequently tongue lick, pinch, and carry around the rat pups. When the researchers tried each of these maneuvers, only the tongue licking (simulated by a paint brush dipped in water and briskly stroked all over the body of the rat pup) restored these values to their normal level. More recently, Schanberg and his colleagues discovered a growth gene that responds to tactile stimulation, suggesting genetic origins of this touch/growth relationship.

Realizing that an exploration of under-the-skin variables including physiology and biochemistry might suggest an underlying mechanism in the human model, we added physiological and biochemical measures to our next study. This study with preterm infants basically confirmed our previous data set. In this sample the stimulated infants showed a 21% greater daily weight gain, were discharged 5 days earlier, showed superior performance on the Brazelton Habituation items, and showed fewer stress behaviors (mouthing, grimacing, and clenched fists) (Scafidi et al., 1990). In addition, we noted that their catecholamines (norepinephrine, epinephrine) had increased across the stimulation period (Kuhn et al., 1991). Although these catecholamines typically increase following stress in the adult, suggesting that an increase is undesirable, an increase during the neonatal period would be considered desirable since there is a normal developmental

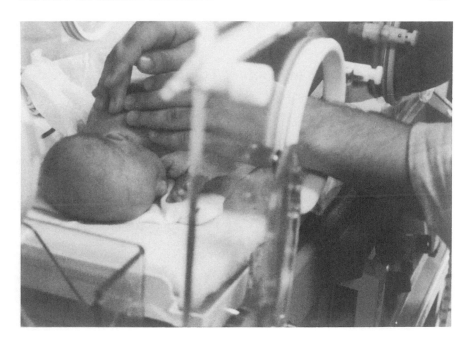

Figure 4.2 Preterm infant being massaged.

increase following birth. Thus, the massage therapy apparently facilitated the normal developmental increase in these catecholamines in the stimulated preterm infants. In the interim we also discovered that their vagal activity increased during massage therapy sessions.

This observation, plus the work of Uvnas-Moberg in Sweden, led us to some ideas about underlying mechanisms. Uvnas-Moberg and her colleagues have reported that stimulating the inside of the mouth of the newborn (and the breast of the mother) led to the increased release of gastrointestinal food absorption hormones such as gastrin and insulin (Uvnas-Moberg et al., 1987). It is conceivable that another form of tactile stimulation, such as the massage therapy on different body parts, could also lead to the release of gastrointestinal food absorption hormones probably stimulated by vagal activity. Thus, we are currently assaying glucose and insulin levels in the heelstick samples of preterm infants, and our preliminary data suggest that the massaged infants are showing elevated levels of insulin.

Most of the research on massage therapy with preterm infants (Figure 4.2) has been conducted with infants who are no longer medically unstable but simply need to gain weight. Until research of this kind is performed with sick preterms, the massage therapy should be confined to those preterm infants who are in the "growing" stage. In addition, other measures might be used, for example, magnetic resonance imaging to assess changes in brain development.

MASSAGE BY MOTHERS AND "GRANDPARENT" VOLUNTEERS

Depressed Mothers Massaging Their Infants

Because we need a cost-effective way to deliver massage therapy to infants, because parents as massage therapists may also benefit from giving massage, and because the parent-infant relationship may improve, we are conducting more and more studies on the effects on teaching parents to administer massage therapy. In a recent study we taught depressed mothers to massage their infants to examine the effects of the massage therapy on the infants' disorganized interaction behavior and their disturbed sleep patterns (Field et al., 1995). Adolescent mothers who have high Beck Depression Inventory scores were recruited for the study shortly after their infants were born. For this study we asked the depressed mothers to perform a 15-minute massage daily for a 2-week period. The results suggested that the following changes occurred for the massaged (as compared to rocked) infants (see Table 4.3): (1) drowsiness and quiet sleep increased immediately following the massage, and activity and crying decreased as might be expected; (2) the infants had lower cortisol levels after the massage; (3) the infants showed improved affect during mother-infant play interactions over the 2-week period; and (4) the infants' depressed mothers perceived their "depressed" infants as being easier to soothe and more sociable. These data on decreased fussiness and more organized sleep suggested that we should conduct studies having parents massage their colicky infants and their infants with sleep disturbances. Thus, we are using the same model for those groups.

Grandparent Volunteers as Massage Therapists

Another cost-effective delivery of massage therapy is via grandparent volunteers. These are not biological grandparents of the children but simply retired people

Table 4.3. Means (and S.D.s) for Sleep/Wake Behaviors During and After Sessions for Massage Therapy and Rocking Groups[*]

	Group				
	Massage Therapy		Rocking		
Variables	During	After	During	After	p
Sleep/Wake Behaviors					
Quiet sleep	4.3 (2)ₐ	48.1 (26)_b	45.9 (21)_b	41.8 (18)_b	.001
Active sleep	0.0 (0)ₐ	4.8 (2)ₐ	0.0 (0)ₐ	0.0 (0)ₐ	NS
Rem sleep	0.0 (0)ₐ	2.9 (2)ₐ	3.1 (2)ₐ	0.0 (0)ₐ	NS
Drowsy	0.8 (0)ₐ	5.3 (3)_b	1.3 (3¹)_b	7.3 (4)_b	.05
Interactive alert	35.6 (16)ₐ	23.6 (14)_b	16.7 (11)_bc	10.9 (6)_c	.05
Active awake	46.2 (26)ₐ	14.3 (9)_b	21.7 (11)_c	29.3 (14)_c	.001
Crying	14.4 (12)ₐ	2.5 (2)_b	8.3 (6)ₐ	10.7 (9)ₐ	.001
Movement	87.7 (39)ₐ	44.1 (21)_b	45.3 (23)_b	56.7 (27)_b	.001
Salvia cortisol[**]	2.1 (1)ₐ	1.4 (1)_b	1.9 (1)_ab	1.5 (1)_b	.05

[*] Different letter subscripts denote significant differences.
[**] Saliva cortisol values taken before and after session.

who prefer the name "grandparent" to elderly volunteers. They belong to an organization of volunteers and have had years of experience with young children. In an ongoing study, grandparent volunteers are being trained to massage neglected and abused infants in a shelter. The study is designed to measure the effects of massage therapy on sexually and physically abused infants living in a nearby shelter, as well as the effects on the volunteer grandparents giving the massage. It is interesting that the other end of the age spectrum, older adults, also experience failure to thrive, probably secondary to touch deprivation. Our objective here was to reduce the grandparents' touch deprivation and the infants' touch deprivation as well to reduce any touch aversions from having been sexually or physically abused. The infants in this study ranged in age from 3 to 18 months, and the volunteers were their primary caregivers in the shelter for the morning hours, so the massage therapy sessions were a structured program integrated into their daily caregiving routine.

In our study on training volunteer grandparents to give neglected and abused infants massage, the preliminary results suggest that when the infants were assessed at the beginning versus the end of treatment the following changes occurred for the infants: (1) drowsiness and quiet sleep increased and activity decreased following the massage; (2) after 1 month of massage therapy, alertness and tracking behaviors increased; and (3) behavior observations suggested increased activity, sociability, and soothability. For the volunteer grandparent massage therapists, a preliminary analysis of the data suggested that (1) the grandparent volunteers reported less anxiety and fewer depression symptoms and an improved mood after receiving the massage; (2) their cortisol levels decreased; (3) their lifestyle improved with more social contacts, fewer trips to the doctor's office, and fewer cups of coffee; and (4) they reported improved self-esteem. These effects appeared to be greater for the grandparents following a month of providing the infants with massage than they were following a month of receiving their own massages. These data suggest the power of massage therapy not only for the infants but for the adult massagers, making it possible to provide infants with cost-effective massage therapy.

We have since discovered many other groups of infants who might benefit from massage therapy, such as those with cancer and spina bifida, as well as adults with different medical conditions who could benefit from providing the therapy. The benefits of massage with normal infants, however, should not be overlooked, as often happens when so many infants have clinical problems needing treatment. The Romanian orphanage infants remind us of the need for physical contact for normal growth and development. The mandate against touching children in our culture (because of potential sexual abuse) may also have severe consequences. And in places where there are no touch taboos, infants thrive (as do their parents) on this pleasurable physical contact.

Acknowledgments

The author would like to thank all of the mothers and infants who participated in this study. This research was supported by NIMH Research Scientist Award (MH00331) and Johnson & Johnson funding to T. F. Correspondence and reprint requests can be sent to Tiffany Field, Department of Pediatrics, University of Miami School of Medicine, P.O. Box 016820, Miami, Florida 33101.

REFERENCES

Auckett, A. D. (1981). *Baby Massage*. New York: Newmarket Press.

Barnard, K. E., & Bee, H. L. (1983). The impact of temporally patterned stimulation on the development of preterm infants. *Child Development 54*, 1156–1167.

Field, T., Grizzle, N., Scafidi, F., Abrams, S., & Richardson, S. (1996). Massage therapy for infants of depressed mothers. *Infant Behavior and Development*. 19, 107–112.

Field, T., Schanberg, S., Scafidi, F., Bower, C., Vega-Lahr, N., Garcia, R., Nystrom, J., & Kuhn, C. M. (1986). Tactile/kinesthetic stimulation effects on preterm neonates. *Pediatrics, 77*, 654–658.

Kuhn, C., Schanberg, S., Field, T., Symanski, R., Zimmerman, E., Scafidi, F., & Roberts, J. (1991). Tactile kinesthetic stimulation effects on sympathetic and adrenocortical function in preterm infants. *Journal of Pediatrics, 119*, 434–440.

McClure, V. S. (1989). *Infant Massage*. New York: Bantam.

Ottenbacher, K. J., Muller, L., Brandt, D., Heintzelman, A., Hojem, P., & Sharpe, P. (1987). The effectiveness of tactile stimulation as a form of early intervention: a quantitative evaluation. *Journal of Developmental and Behav Pediatr, 8*, 68–76.

Rausch, P. B. (1981). Neurophysicalogical development in premature infants following stimulation. *Developmental Psychology, 13*, 69–76.

Rice, R. D. (1977). Neurophysiological development in premature infants following stimulation. *Developmental Psychology, 13*, 69–76.

Scafifi, F., & Field, T. (1996). Massage therapy improves behavior in neonates born to HIV positive mothers. *Journal of Pediatric Psychology, 21, 889–897*.

Scafidi, F., Field, T., Schanberg, S., Bauer, C., Tucci, K., Roberts, J., Morrow, C. & Kuhn, C. M. (1990). Massage stimulates growth in preterm infants: a replication. *Infant Behavior and Development*. 13, 167–188.

Schanberg, S., & Field, T. (1988). Maternal deprivation and supplemental stimulation. In T. Field, P. McCabe, & N. Scheniderman (Eds.), *Stress and Coping Across Development*. Hillsdale, NJ: Lawrence Erlbaum.

Solkoff, N., & Matuszak, D. (1975). Tactile stimulation and behavioral development among low-birthweight infants. *Child Psychiatry and Human Development, 6*, 33–37.

Uvnas-Moberg, K., Widstrom, A. M., Marchine, G., & Windberg, J. (1987). Release of GI hormone in mothers and infants by sensory stimulation. *Acta Paediatrica Scandinavia, 76*, 851–860.

Wheeden, A., Scafidi, F. A., Field, T., Ironson, G., & Valdeon, C. (1993) Massge effects on cocaine-exposed preterm neonates. *Journal of Developmental & Behavioral Pediatrics* 14, 318–322.

White, J. L., & LaBarba, R. C. (1976). The effects of tactile and kinesthetic stimulation on neonatal development in the premature infant. *Developmental Psychobiology, 6* 569–577.

5

VESTIBULAR STIMULATION AS A NEURODEVELOPMENTAL INTERVENTION WITH PRETERM INFANTS: FINDINGS AND NEW METHODS OF REVALUATING INTERVENTION EFFECTS

ANNELIESE F. KORNER

With the recent technological advances in neonatology that have resulted in the survival of an increasing number of very young preterm infants, behavioral scientists have become concerned about the quality of life in neonatal intensive care units (NICUs). This concern has led to many different in-hospital intervention studies over the last 20 years, with varied rationales, and methodological approaches. The choices depended largely on whether preterm infants were viewed as babies deprived of the many forms of stimulation prevalent in a natural home environment or as infants deprived of forms of stimulation highly prevalent in *in utero*. In the absence of solid research evidence, it seems to make sense to provide compensatory forms of stimulation similar to those prevailing *in utero* to very young preterm infants and to expose babies near term to forms of stimulation prevalent in natural home environments. (For further discussion of these issues, see Korner, 1987.)

In our own intervention research, we decided to intervene with *young* preterm infants to determine whether a change in the infants' incubator environment might improve their clinical or developmental course. In this in-hospital intervention, the aim was to develop infants functioning well enough to become more gratifying partners in their earliest relationship with their parents.

All the issues one typically faces when setting up experimental studies involving stimulation were inherent in ours. The options are many and the underlying theoretical issues are manifold. For example, one might ask what forms of stimulation might be developmentally the most relevant at different postconceptional ages. One might also ask whether the sensory system utilized in providing stimulation to preterm infants at any given age makes a difference. Should one choose a sensory system whose functioning is well established, or is about to begin to function, or whose functioning will mature only at a later time? Is the patterning or the rhythm of the stimulation important? should rhythms be used that have some biological revelance or are arbitrary choices just as beneficial? If biological relevant rhythms are chosen, should one adopt maternal types of temporal biological rhythms, or is it perhaps more appropriate to reinforce the infants' mature behaviors, or should an attempt be made to entrain infants into biological rhythms that, in the course of maturation, they will develop by themselves?

This chapter is divided into two parts: the first part addresses the rationale for our choices for the intervention and summarizes the results of our intervention studies. The second part discusses new methods of assessing intervention effects.

THE INTERVENTION

History, Rationale and Description of Our Intervention Research

The choices in our approach to intervention were guided by the results of a 10-year series of developmental studies with full-term infants and rat pups (Korner & Grobstein, 1966; Korner & Thoman, 1970, 1972; Thoman & Korner, 1971; Gregg, Haffner, & Korner, 1976). In the course of these studies, my colleagues and I found that young infants are exquisitely responsive to vestibular-proprioceptive stimulation. Langworthy (1933), Hooker (1952), Humphrey (1965), and Gottlieb (1971) pointed to the early functional maturity of the vestibular system, which made good ontogenetic sense to us. Considering this evidence in the literature and the results of our developmental studies, I concluded that it might be beneficial to provide compensatory movement stimulation to young preterm infants, who experience this type of stimulation prenatally but not in incubators.

The rationale for this type of intervention was also underscored by reports from the animal literature, which suggested that deprivation of movement stimulation may lead to major developmental deficits. For example, Erway (1975), whose work focused on otolith function in mice, concluded that "deficiency of vestibular input either for reasons of congenital defect or for lack of motion stimulation, may impair the early development and integrating capacities of the brain, especially that of the cerebellum." Mason's work (1968, 1979) with non-human primates underscored this conclusion and pointed to the fundamental importance of movement stimulation for the intactness of early development. Like Harlow (1958), Mason reared infant monkeys in isolation on surrogate mothers. While Harlow produced highly abnormal monkeys who engaged in autistic-like self-mutilating and rocking behavior, Mason offset the most severe developmental deficits in Harlow's monkeys by providing monkeys in isolation with *swinging* surrogate mothers.

The most gentle way I could think of to provide compensatory movement stimulation to preterm infants was through waterbeds. I want to stress that our intent in providing waterbeds to preterm infants was *not* to simulate the intra-uterine environment, which is neither possible in a qualitative sense nor necessarily desirable. All we intended to provide was gentle movement stimulation, which is highly prevalent *in utero*. We also hoped that the fluid support provided by the waterbeds might preserve the fragile skin of very young preterm infants and might reduce the incidence of oblong, oddly shaped heads so frequently seen in preterms, and so worrisome to their parents.

Stimulus Characteristics of the Infant Waterbeds

In 1972, we began developing the infant waterbeds that could function in three different modes: as a plain waterbed highly responsive to the infant's own movements and the movements generated by the caregiver and as a waterbed that gently oscillates either continuously or intermittently. The waterbeds that provide slight containment for the infants were adapted to all the intensive-care contingencies. The thermal environment created by the waterbeds was thoroughly investigated in collaborative studies with the Stanford Thermal Engineering Department. Because the waterbed is just above the incubator heater, its temperature is maintained at 2°C above the ambient temperature inside the isolette. We inferred from this that the waterbed may help the temperature regulation of very young preterm infants kept in very warm incubators. When used outside the incubator, or when the isolette is at relatively low temperatures, *it is absolutely necessary to use 1/2 inch of foam to insulate the waterbed from the baby* to prevent infant heat loss.

In making decisions regarding the frequency, direction, amplitude, and rhythm of the oscillations, I tried to avoid arbitrary choices. Instead, I chose according to clinical, biological, or experiental relevance. My colleagues and I chose head-to-foot oscillations because studies in the neonatal literature suggested that this direction of motion may benefit infants' respiratory efforts (Lee, 1954; Millen & Davies, 1946). Because many infants would remain on the waterbed for long periods of time, we decided on oscillations that measure no more than 2.4 millimeters in amplitude at the surface of the waterbed without an infant in place. These oscillations are so gentle they can barely be seen.

In deciding on the frequency or the rhythm of the oscillations, I felt it was safest to provide oscillations in the temporal pattern of maternal biological rhythms, because such rhythms would probably not interfere with the developing organization of the infants' own biological rhythms. I was influenced in this decision by Dreyfus-Brisac's (1974) hypothesis that the behavior and sleep of preterm infants are fragmented because these babies lack the regulatory influences of maternal biological rhythms. The work of several investigators, such as Sterman (1967), Jeannerod (1969), Hofer (1975, 1976) and Bertini, Antonioli, and Gambi (1978), also suggests such influences. For example, Sterman and Jeannerod independently showed a strong relationship between maternal sleep stages and intrauterine fetal activity. In the light of this evidence in the literature, we thought that oscillations in the pattern of maternal biological rhythms might enhance infants' functioning. We thus chose the slightly irregular continuous oscillations in the rhythm in the lower range of the average maternal resting respirations (12–14 pulses per minute) in the 3rd trimester of pregnancy (Good-lin, 1972). For the intermittent oscillations, we chose the same irregular rhythm with on-off intervals in the temporal pattern of the basic rest-activity cycle as described by Kleitman (1969).

Figure 5.1 is a photograph of our waterbed and of the compact microprocessor that generates the oscillations. The following is a brief summary of the findings of six randomized, controlled waterbed studies conducted by our laboratory.

Study 1

We began with a study designed to test whether changing the infants' environment on a 24-hour basis by placing them on waterbeds was a safe procedure (Korner et al., 1975). Twenty-one relatively healthy preterm infants, ranging in gestational ages between 27 and 34 weeks, were randomly assigned to experimental and control groups. The groups did not differ significantly in their gestational ages, birthweights or health status. The infants in the experimental group were each placed on the continuously, though irregularly, oscillating waterbed before they were 6 days old. They remained in the experimental condition for 1 week. The data were collected from the physicians' and nurses' daily progress notes, including mean daily apical pulse rates and respiration rates, mean and ranges of daily temperature, weight, incidence of emesis, concentrations of oxygen administered, and incidence of apnea. From these notes the clinical progress of the two groups was compared.

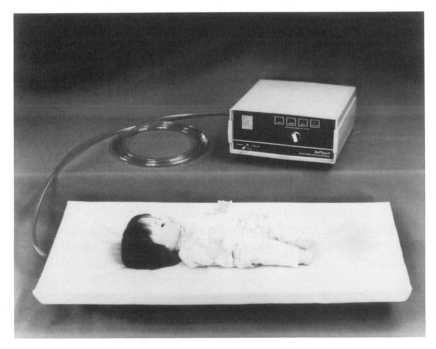

Figure 5.1. Preterm infant waterbed with oscillator.

The results of this study showed that none of the infants' vital signs was significantly affected by the waterbeds, nor did weight changes or the incidence of emesis differ in the two groups. However, one highly significant difference was found between the two groups, which is shown in Figure 5.2. The infants in the experimental group had significantly fewer apneas as indicated by the apnea alarms. The incidence of apnea did not differ significantly in the two groups at the beginning of the study, but as soon as the infants in the experimental group were placed on the waterbed, their apneas tended to level off, whereas the apneas of infants in the control group increased, the more usual course when apnea begins shortly after birth.

Study 2

Since apnea can cause brain damage, it was essential to determine whether our finding could be replicated. We decided to put this question to the test in a collaborative polygraphic study with Dr. C. Guilleminault from the Stanford Sleep Disorder Clinic (Korner, et al., 1978). The sleep and respiratory patterns of a small group of preterm infants who were preselected for having apnea of prematurity were polygraphically recorded for a 24-hour period. The 24-hour recordings were divided into 4 time blocks, with the infant placed on the waterbed during two 6-hour periods. To avoid an order effect, the sequence of the experimental and control conditions was alternated.

We confirmed our previous finding that apneas significantly decreased while the infants were on the oscillating waterbed. This was true of all types of apneas, including short 10-second ones and longer ones, as well as obstructive and central apneas. The most consistent reductions occurred in the apneas significantly reduced in our previous study, namely, those that were long enough to trip the monitor alarms. Figure 5.3 displays these results. The most severe types of apnea, as defined by their association with slowing of the heart rate to below 80 beats

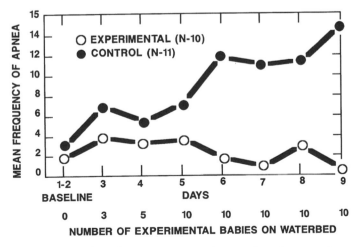

Figure 5.2. Comparison between experimental and control groups in the mean daily apnea incidence.

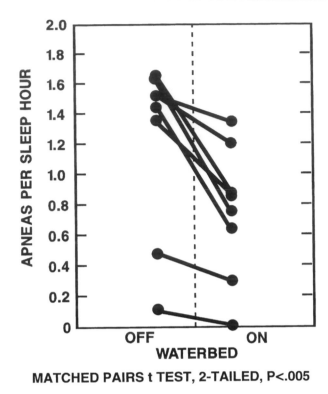

Figure 5.3. Apnea monitor alarms per sleep hour, off and on the oscillating waterbed.

per minute, were most sharply reduced, at least in 7 of the 8 babies. However, one infant's response ran completely counter to that of the group (Figure 5.4).

We found out later that this infant was not a typical case of apnea of prematurity, and that this infant was not unique. Highly unstable infants who have major endocrine, neurological, or cardiopulmonary problems or infants treated with theophylline are not apt to respond to waterbeds with apnea reduction. We concluded from this study and from subsequent observations that this treatment approach probably benefits primarily those infants who have a diagnosis of uncomplicated apnea of prematurity.

Studies 3, 4, and 5

Because waterbeds were used in many quarters in the 1970s, we wanted to ascertain whether waterbeds had any effects on the infants' sleep and wake states and on their motility. To this end, we undertook three studies:

1. In this study, 17 preterm infants on a regimen of theophylline for apnea of prematurity were recruited to determine whether slow irregular waterbed oscillations (9 per minute) could augment their sleep, which commonly is sharply decreases as a function of any caffeine-type drug (Korner, Ruppel, & Rho, 1982).

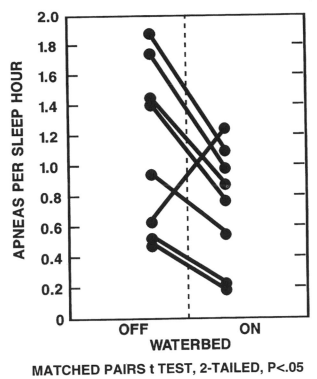

APNEAS PER SLEEP HOUR

OFF ON
WATERBED

MATCHED PAIRS t TEST, 2-TAILED, P<.05

Figure 5.4. Apneas > 10 seconds per sleep hour with bradycardia below 80 beats per minute.

2. Twelve very healthy preterm infants were assessed on and off the waterbeds that oscillated intermittently in the temporal pattern of a maternal biological rhythm (Edelman, Kraemer, & Korner, 1982).

3. This study included 52 healthy preterm infants who were recruited to compare the differential efficacy of nonoscillating, continuously, and intermittently oscillating waterbeds in enhancing sleep and in soothing preterms (Korner et al., 1990).

In each study, the infants served as their own control on and off the waterbed. The method of observation was the same in each study: the infants' sleep-wake states and the quality of their movements were observed in 10-second epochs. In each study, the infants were in the experimental and control condition for four days and were observed on the 3rd and 4th day in each condition. On each of the four days they were observed, the infants' states were assessed for 100 minutes each.

The results of these 3 studies were very consistent: in each study, quiet sleep significantly increased and crying significantly decreased while the infants were on the waterbeds. This replicated finding generalized over 3 independent samples of different types of preterm infants. Additionally, the infants on theophylline and the 52 healthy preterms had significantly reduced sleep latencies, less restlessness during sleep, fewer state changes, and unsmooth and jittery movements. In comparing the efficacy of the 3 different types of waterbeds, irritability was reduced the most on the continuously oscillating waterbed.

Study 6

We also began to systematically investigate what we had originally set out to do, namely, to study the effects of waterbeds on the neurobehavioral development of preterm infants (Korner, Schneider, & Forrest, 1983). The 56 subjects in this longitudinal study were randomly assigned to experimental and control groups before they were 4 days old. For homogeneity of diagnosis, all infants who were on ventilators for severe respiratory distress were selected. The infants ranged in gestational ages between 22 and 32 weeks. Birthweights, gestational ages, and Apgar scores did not differ significantly between the two groups.

To measures the differential maturity of the two groups at the end of the intervention, we developed a new, more fine-grained neurobehavioral assessment than was available in 1977. Twenty infants were available for final evaluation when they were between 34 and 35 weeks postconceptional age. The birth characteristics of these infants were very similar to those of the babies who originally had been randomly assigned to groups. The infants in the experimental group were removed from the waterbeds at least 48 hours prior to being assessed. All infants were then examined by a pediatrician trained in neurology (T. Forrest), who did not know which babies belonged in the control or the experimental groups.

The results of this study showed that the infants in the experimental group demonstrated significantly more mature motor behavior, were significantly less irritable, were more than twice as often in the visually alert inactive state, and performed significantly better attending and pursuing inanimate and animate visual and auditory stimuli. This pilot study thus suggested that compensatory movement stimulation as provided by gently oscillating waterbeds likely enhances the neurobehavioral development of preterm infants.

Clinical Uses of the Nonoscillating Waterbed

Nonoscillating waterbeds have frequently been requested by the nurses and medical staff to alleviate a variety of clinical conditions. Clinicians have reported to us that the waterbeds have been very helpful in the care of very young preterm infants who weighed no more than 1 to 2 pounds and who were kept in very hot incubators. They also reported that these warm beds stabilized these infants' temperature and that the fluid support preserved their fragile skin. According to clinicians, the nonoscillating waterbeds have also been helpful in reducing the discomfort of infants with spina bifida, osteogenesis imperfecta, disseminated herpes, and other types of severe skin conditions. Further, the nonoscillating waterbeds were found useful for infants recovering from abdominal surgery, as these infants could not be turned prone, and for infants on a regimen of parenteral nutrition for severe emaciation. In any clinical condition in which pressure points to the skin or the skeletal structure are to be avoided, waterbeds

seem to have beneficial effects. In line with this rationale, waterbeds have frequently been requested to diminish the incidence of scaphocephalic heads so
commonly seen in preterm infants.

For all the above conditions, the use of the nonoscillating waterbed is sufficient
and, in most of these conditions, probably is preferable to the oscillating waterbed. This is especially true in the treatment of tiny, fragile babies or of any
infants in whom even the slightest passive movement might cause discomfort.

Practical, Clinical, and Theoretical Implications of our Intervention Studies

One may conclude from our studies that it makes clinical sense to try the oscillating waterbed for infants with uncomplicated mild apnea of prematurity. If
an infant fails to respond, other treatments should of course be instituted. Judg-
ing from the findings of three of our studies, it also makes clinical sense to use
waterbeds to enhance sleep and to reduce irritability in preterm infants. Although both the oscillating and nonoscillating waterbeds created these effects,
clearly the oscillating waterbeds are more effective in reducing irritability. Oscillating waterbeds should therefore be used for this purpose with very irritable
infants. Although there were strong indications that waterbeds oscillating in a
maternal biological rhythm enhanced the neurobehavioral development of preterm infants, this finding is based on only 1 study that we have not tried to
replicate. A longitudinal study, such as we conducted, that assesses the effects of
compensatory movement stimulation on the neurobehavioral development of
preterm infants would be highly desirable. For such a developmental study, it
might be preferable to use intermittent oscillations to minimize the possibility of
the infants' habituating to the oscillations and to provide an environment that
exposes the infants to a biological rhythm involving both periods of activity and
rest.

After some of our articles appeared in the literature, many other types of
waterbeds for preterm infants began to be produced. Most of these devices are
used in the clinical care of preterms and, to my knowledge, have not been
systematically tested for their safety or their effects. We have heard some nurseries use waterbeds inside or outside incubators without appropriate insulation.
This places preterm infants at great risk for hypothermia, which causes, among
other problems, failure to gain weight. On the other hand, heating devices are
frequently used to warm waterbeds. These also pose certain problems because
little is known about the optimal temperature for an infant waterbed. In particular, an overly warm temperature can cause apnea (Daily, Klaus, & Meyer,
1969; Perlstein, Edwards, & Sutherland, 1970). It is clear that the safest way to
protect preterm infants from adverse thermal conditions is to insulate the waterbed with half an inch of foam. This fact, unfortunately, is not widely appre-
ciated.

Differently constructed waterbeds have also been used in a few research studies by other investigators, some based on the assumption that the waterbeds
would produce the same effects as ours. Such assumptions are unwarranted.

Waterbeds can be soft or hard, insulated or not, provide containment or not, and oscillate regularly, irregularly, or intermittently, gently or vigorously, at high or at low frequencies or not at all. Yet it has been widely assumed that all types of waterbeds, merely by virtue of being waterbeds, will have the same effects. Thus, for example, "bumpbeds," which are not waterbeds at all, have been used on the assumption that intermittent, rather vigorous jerks would reduce apnea. Probably the worst example of sloppy analogous reasoning was perpetrated by a company that prepared a brochure on "apnea therapy" that copied our articles on this subject, from which the company concluded that its device, which produced undulating displacement of air, would be much more convenient to use for the same purpose. Generally, one cannot naively assume that different equipment providing movement stimulation, or different waterbeds, or different research protocols will produce the same effects. The effects will differ depending on the specific stimulus characteristics of the waterbeds, the specific research protocols used, and the populations studied. Any one of these factors will affect outcomes and replication of the findings. This issue is well illustrated in the early literature with animal models. Very minor changes in the kind, quality, quantity, or interval of stimulation can lead to major differences in outcome (e.g., Brown & Martin, 1974 Schanberg, Evoniuk, & Kuhn, 1984). The implication is, of course, that the safety and the treatment effects of differently designed waterbeds need to be separately and systematically investigated through randomized, controlled studies.

As some of our articles appeared in the literature, there were several spinoffs from our work that I consider unfortunate. For one, waterbeds have been produced for home use with postterm infants, where there is a huge market. Through the years, dozens of parents have called me to find out where to purchase a waterbed so as not to deprive their new baby of "every advantage." I uniformly have cautioned these parents against using waterbeds because, unlike preterm infants who are continuously attended by nursing staff, infants at home are not watched continuously, particularly during the night. Conceivably, infants placed in the prone on a loosely filled waterbed may experience difficulty in lifting their heads from the surface of the bed. Also, even small amounts of water from a leak could potentially present a drowning hazard. Aside from these considerations, nothing is known about the developmental effects of waterbed flotation on the sleep and the motor development of older infants. Because young babies lie in bed much of the time during the first few months of life, it is imperative that systematic randomized studies document whether prolonged waterbed flotation has beneficial, deleterious, or no effects on the development of postterm infants. Moreover, while there is a theoretical rationale for providing preterms with compensatory vestibular-proprioceptive stimulation because they are largely deprived of this developmentally important form of stimulation when growing to term in incubators, there is no such rationale for postterm infants, who usually experience ample movement stimulation in the course of ordinary child care.

Because our studies have shown a reduction of apnea and bradycardia in infants with a diagnosis of apnea of prematurity, the question has frequently been raised about whether it would be helpful to provide oscillating waterbeds for SIDS-prone young children. To conduct a scientific study to determine whether sleep apnea is reduced in these children would be very difficult because fortunately these infants are quite rare. Certainly it would be dangerous to rely in any way on an oscillating waterbed to protect a SIDS-prone child without, at the same time, using the usual safeguards such as an apnea monitor.

NEW METHODS FOR ASSESSING INTERVENTION EFFECTS

Neurobehavioral Assessment of the Preterm Infant

Development of the Neurobehavioral Assessment of the Preterm Infant (NAPI) began in 1977 in the context of our longitudinal intervention study described before (Korner et al., 1983). When we found that the preliminary version of the NAPI discriminated significantly between randomly assigned groups of experimental and control infants, that its test-retest reliability was high in a number of important functions and that its interobserver reliability was readily established, we decided that it might be helpful to further develop this procedure for general use.

In developing this instrument, we started from the premise that the most relevant and important goal of any intervention would be to facilitate the normality of the infants' developmental course so that their ultimate development and maturity would not be too different from that of normal full-term newborns (Korner, 1987). Thus, to measure the effects of an intervention, the prime objective of an assessment should be to measure the functional maturity of randomly assigned experimental and control groups of preterm infants (Korner, 1989). There were no such instruments available in 1977, except the ones by Saint-Anne Dagassies (1966) and by Amiel-Tison (1968), which, however, characterized infant performance only in age intervals of 2 weeks. Because, it seemed unrealistic to expect that experimental and control groups would differ in functional maturity in excess of 2 weeks, we felt we should develop a procedure that could reveal more subtle differences in performance. In line with our goal of developing a maturity assessment, we limited our selection of test items to those that promised to show developmental changes over time, as suggested by the literature. Also, we developed a numerical scoring system in which all item scores ranged from the least mature to the most mature responses. Further, we made it our first priority to include in the assessment only conceptually and clinically meaningful test items, which then were tested for their psychometric soundness. Thus, before incorporating any items or clusters into the procedure, we assessed their test-retest reliability, redundancy and developmental validity.

After our pilot study (Korner et al., 1983), we developed the NAPI in its present form (Korner & Thom, 1990) in 3 phases.

In Phase 1, in which the pilot version of the test was revised, conceptual clusters that had face validity were then formed, and a series of statistical procedures were used to ascertain the test-retest reliability of the clusters and test items. This was followed by assessment of the developmental validity of those clusters and test items that had a minimum test-retest reliability of 0.6. This phase of test development included 179 preterm infants (Korner et al., 1987).

Phase 2 was a validation and replication study with an independent cohort of 290 infants (Korner et al., 1991).

Phase 3 assessed the clinical validity and sensitivity of the test. For this purpose, we developed a new, simple to score neonatal medical index (NMI). This study included 471 preterm infants (Korner et al., 1994).

Subjects

To recruit as representative a sample of preterm infants as was feasible, infants were recruited from both tertiary and intermediate care nurseries from 4 San Francisco Bay Area hospitals and 1 nursery in Portland, Oregon. Also, in order to generate results that would be representative of preterm infants in general, exclusion criteria for the subjects in the two independent cohorts were kept to an absolute minimum. Excluded were infants whose gestational age estimates were discrepant by more than 2 weeks. The 4 gestational age estimates used were the mother's and obstetrician's dates of confinement (EDC), the Ballard Assessment (Ballard, Novak, & Driver, 1979), the infant's head circumference, and, when available, an ultrasound examination. To further reduce potential errors in gestational age estimates, the most commonly available estimates (EDC and Ballard) of the eligible infants were averaged. The only other infants excluded were those who had diagnoses suggesting central nervous system damage, such as known Grade III and IV intraventricular hemorrhages, persistent seizures, disseminated herpes, or severe asphyxia at birth. Data for the three phases of the test's development were collected between 1983 and 1989. Informed consent for the infants' inclusion in the studies was obtained from one or both parents.

Description of the NAPI

The NAPI is applicable to medically stable infants from 32 weeks conceptional age to term. Because preterm infants have a relatively small neurobehavioral repertoire, most of the test items in the assessment necessarily overlap with those used in other neurobehavioral examinations. The NAPI differs primarily in the developmental rationale underlying the choice of the test items (infants' responses had to show significant age progressions on longitudinal testing), in the scoring system, and in the statistical approach to establishing the test's reliability and developmental validity described before. In fact, the psychometric soundness of the test items and clusters was made a *precondition* to their inclusion in the assessment. Also, the exclusion of aversive maneuvers, such as the Moro and the pin prick, differed from other procedures. Further, we decided to use a strictly invariant sequence of item presentation designed to bring about the behavioral states most likely to elicit the best possible responses from preterm infants. Even though we were keenly aware that infant states strongly influence their responses (Korner, 1972), we found empirically that, with young preterm infants, the requirement of a predetermined state before administering each item was not feasible. An attempt to achieve the appropriate predetermined states through various rousing and soothing maneuvers would have greatly prolonged the examination, fatigued the infant, or failed altogether. For this reason, we chose to build into the assessment a standard sequence of rousing, soothing, and alerting items that maximized the chance of testing the various functions in appropriate states and minimized the need to intervene with some infants more than with others. To illustrate, we try to rouse the infants who, for the most part, are asleep 45 minutes before the next feeding, when typically the assessments are made, by administering the scarf sign and the arm and leg recoil. Items like the Popliteal angle, ventral suspension, head lift, and spontaneous crawling can then be administered in more awake states. All the infants are then swaddled to calm those who have become irritable. The rotation test is then administered in preparation for modified Brazelton (1973) orientation items, as we had found in earlier studies (Korner & Grobstein, 1966; Korner & Thoman, 1970) that the vestibular-proprioceptive stimulation entailed in moving the infant predictably produces visual alertness. This approach prevented the examination from becoming a different procedure for each infant. This strategy also provided the opportunity to systematically study the age changes in the infants' states in response to a standard sequence of identical events (Korner et al., 1988).

Our methodological and statistical approach resulted in a relatively brief and gentle instrument consisting of 7 reliable and developmentally valid clusters or single-item neurobehavioral dimensions that represent a conceptually and clinically meaningful spectrum of preterm infant functions. These are the dimensions, which contain 27 subitems, scorable on 3-to 9-point scales:

1. Motor development and vigor
2. Scarf signs
3. Popliteal angle
4. Alertness and orientation
5. Irritability
6. Vigor of crying
7. Percentage asleep ratings

Additionally, the procedure includes a number of summary rating scales involving the quality of spontaneous movements, of visual behavior, and of crying, as well as infant reactions to the handling and stimulation provided by the examination. The latter addresses the issue of how infants vary in their excitation management (Korner, 1996).

Use of the NAPI as an Instrument for Evaluating the Effects of Interventions

Because the NAPI was specifically developed to assess the effects of an intervention (see study 6, Korner et al., 1983), it was constructed to measure whether any behavioral intervention enhances, facilitates, and solidifies the infants' developmental course? The procedure thus is ideally suited to measure intervention effects either on groups or individuals, because it assesses the relative *maturity* of infant functioning. Provided that experimental and control groups were comparable before the intervention in weight, gestational age, and so on, one can use the normative guidelines that are a part of the procedure to determine whether the experimental group functions at a more mature level. In assessing the effects of remedial intervention on individual infants who early on showed *consistent* developmental lags in certain functions, one can determine through longitudinal testing whether there is catch-up in performance in these functions.

The NAPI can also be used for additional purposes, such as these:

1. To study the stability of individual differences in developmentally changing preterm infants (e.g., Korner et al., 1989).
2. To gain basic knowledge regarding the nature and sequence of preterm infants' behavioral development (e.g., Korner et al., 1988).
3. To generate normative data that describe the gradual unfolding of the behavioral repertoire of preterm infants as they grow to term (e.g., Korner & Thom, 1990).
4. To monitor the developmental progress of individual infants.
5. To demonstrate to parents their infant's developmental progress over repeated examinations (e.g., Constantinou & Korner, 1993).
6. To asses differences in functioning between full-term drug-addicted infants and controls.

NAPI Training

Potentially, any professional caring for or studying premature infants in an NICU is eligible to become a NAPI examiner. Training consists of two major and equally important components-achieving reliability of administering the assessment and achieving reliability in scoring the test items, Prior experience in handling young infants, knowledge of the medical problems and physiological stress reactions frequently seen in preterm infants, and familiarity with infant behavioral states are essential.

The NAPI kit (Korner & Thom, 1990) contains among other things a training videotape and an instruction manual. To become a qualified examiner, one must repeatedly view the training tape to learn exactly how the examination should be administering. Especially important is to learn the flow and sequence of administering the test items, as well as the standard, slow-paced, gentle method of handing an infant. Adherence to the standard examination technique is essential, not only to minimize infant stress reactions but also to elicit infant responses within the range of those obtained during the standardization of the assessment. The training period includes practice and scoring the examination on a minimum of 20 preterm infants of various ages, with re-viewing the training tape, and re-reading the manual between assessments as needed. To complete the training, the reliability of administration and scoring should be evaluated by a qualified teacher of the NAPI in one-on-one training sessions.

The Neonatel Medical Index (NMI)

The NMI was developed to test the clinical sensitivity of the NAPI (Korner et al., 1994). In this clinical validation study, the question was whether the NAPI differentiated the performance of infants who had severe medical complications from that of infants who had an uncomplicated medical course. Because severe illness usually weakens an organism, we hypothesized that test items requiring infant vigor and strength would be affected by prior medical complications, whereas other functions might be unaffected. The results of this study clearly supported this hypothesis in that infant scores in motor development and vigor, irritability, and vigor of crying significantly decreased in infants with a history of severe illness. The discriminatory power of the NMI was not only seen in this study but was confirmed in a predictive external validation study (Korner et al., 1993). In this study, we had the opportunity to use the preexisting data of the 8-site Infant Health and Development Program (1990). The results of this study indicated that the NMI was predictive of later cognitive and motor development and that in infants born at <1,500 g, the effects of neonatal medical complications persisted at least to 3 years of age.

Description of the NMI

In developing the NMI, we sought to produce a simple classification system that, at the time of hospital discharge, would summarize in bold strokes the medical course of preterm infants. The NMI was designed to measure how ill the infants were during their hospital stay, rather than being based on a complete inventory of all the different complications and symptoms the infants had experienced. The few components of the NMI were selected because of their clinical salience and their ready availability on brief chart reviews.

The NMI classifications range from I to V, with I describing preterm infants free of significant past medical problems and V characterizing infants with the most serious complications. This NMI classification is based on two overarching principles: (1) infants with birthweights >1,000 g who experienced no major medical complications are assigned NMI classifications of I or II, and infants born at <1,000 g or heavier babies who had experienced major medical complications receive NMI classifications of III, IV, or V; (2) the need and duration of mechanically assisted ventilation required (ventilatory care or intubation on continuous positive airway pressure [CPAP], or mask or nasal CPAP). The choice of the assisted ventilation classification principle was based on the rationale that, with a few exceptions, the duration of assisted ventilation would be dictated by the length and severity of illness or complications.

The following are the criteria for classifying the NMI:

    I. Birthweight >1,000 g; free of respiratory distress and other major medical complications; no oxygen required; absence of apnea or bradycardia; allowable complications are benign heart murmur and need for phototherapy.

   II. Birthweight >1,000 g; assisted ventilation for 48 hours or less and/or oxygen required 1 or more days; no Periventriculer leukomalacia-intraventricular hemorrhage (PVH-IVH); allowable complications are occasional apnea and/or bradycardia not requiring theophylline or related drugs: Patent ductus arterious (PDA) not requiring medication such as indomethacin.

III. Assisted ventilation for 3–14 days and/or any conditions listed under III below.

IV. Assisted ventilation for 15–28 days and/or any conditions listed under IV below.

V. Assisted ventilation 29 days or more and/or any conditions listed under V below.

Several conditions require a classification of III, IV, or V, regardless of length of time on assisted ventilation:

III. Birthweight <1,000 g; PVH-IVH grade I or II; apnea and/or bradycardia requiring theophylline; patent ductus arterious requiring indomethacin; hyperbilirubinemia requiring exchange transfusion.

IV. Resuscitation needed for apnea or bradycardia while on theophylline; major surgery including PDA (exclude hernias, testicular torsion).

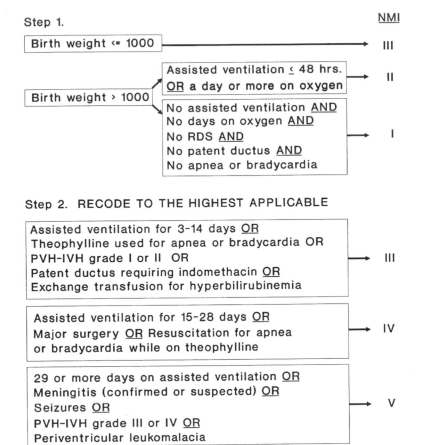

Figure 5.5. Instructions for computing NMI. (Screen for criteria in the order given.)

V. Meningitis confirmed or suspected; seizures; PVH-IVH grade III or IV; periventricular leukomalacia.

All of the above criteria for NMI classifications apply to appropriate, small-, and large-for-gestational age infants. Figure 5.5 displays the algorithm with a set of instructions to compute the NMI. By using the above medical terms, it is possible to retrieve from the infants' medical charts the information needed for the algorithm and the NMI calculations.

Use of the NMI as an Instrument for Evaluating the Effects of Intervention

Although the NMI was originally developed to test the clinical validity of the NAPI, it could be used as an outcome measure that assesses the clinical effects of different interventions. Provided that experimental and control groups start out with comparable weights and gestational ages, one can ascertain in simple numerical terms whether the infants in the experimental group had a more benign medical course during their hospital stay than did controls.

In addition to using the NMI as an outcome measure for intervention studies, it is currently being used by several investigators to describe the characteristics of their study populations. Potentially, the NMI could also predict postterm developmental or medical outcomes. Such a study is now in progress.

SUMMARY

In this chapter, the findings of 6 randomized, controlled experimental studies were described in which compensatory vestibular-proprioceptive stimulation was provided to preterm infants in the form of waterbed flotation. The first study in this series showed that our waterbeds were safe to use in the care of preterm infants and that infants placed on waterbeds had significantly fewer apneas and bradycardias than did a randomly assigned control group. A second study in which the infants served as their own controls, and in which their respiration and heart rates were polygraphically recorded for a 24-hour period, confirmed that apnea and bradycardia significantly decreased during waterbed flotation. In 3 studies the infants' sleep-wake states were monitored on and off the waterbeds. In each of the studies, quiet sleep significantly increased and irritability significantly decreased while the infants were on the waterbeds. In a longitudinal study, the neurobehavioral development of infants growing to term on waterbeds was significantly more mature than that of a randomly assigned control group. The theoretical, clinical, and practical implications of these studies were discussed.

In the course of these studies, we developed two new methods for evaluating the effects of interventions suitable for general use: (1) the NAPI, whose reliability and developmental and clinical validity were thoroughly investigated, and (2) the NMI, which can be used to ascertain in simple numerical terms significant differences in the medical course of experimental and control groups.

Acknowledgments

The research described in this chapter was supported by the Stanford Center for the Study of Families, Children and Youth and by grant RR-81 from the General Clinical Center's Program of the Division of Human Resources, National Institutes of Health.

Figure 5.2 was reprinted with permission from an article by Korner, A. F., Kraemer, H. C. Haffner, M. E., et al., Effects of waterbed flotation on premature infants: a pilot study, *Pediatrics* 1975, 56, 361–367.

Figure 5.3 was reprinted with permission from an article by Korner, A. F., Guilleminault, C., Van den Hoede, J., et al., Reduction of sleep apnea and bradycardia in preterm infants on oscillating waterbeds: a controlled polygraphic study, *Pediatrics* 1978, 61, 528–533.

The criteria and algorithm for scoring the NMI were reprinted with permission from an article by Korner, A. F., Stevenson, D. K., Kraemer, H. C., Spiker, D., Scott, D. T., Constantinou, J., and Dimiceli, S., Prediction of the development of the low birth weight preterm infants by a new neonatal medical index, *J Dev Behav Pediatr* 1993, 14, 106–111 (copyright holder Williams and Wilkins).

REFERENCES

Amiel-Tison, C. (1968). Neurological evaluation of the maturity of new born infants. *Arch Dis Childhood, 43*, 89–93.

Ballard, J. L., Novak, K. K., & Driver, M. (1979). A simplified score for assessment of fetal maturation of newly born infants. *J Pediatr, 95(5)*, 769–774.

Bertini, M., Antonioli, M., & Gambi, D. (1978). Intrauterine mechanisms of synchronization: in search of the first dialogue. *Totus Homo, 10(8))*, 73–91.

Brazelton, T. B. (1973). Neonatal Behavioral Assessment Scale. *Clin Dev Med, 50*. Philadelphia: J. B. Lippincott.

Brown, G. M., & Martin, J. B. (1974). Corticosterone, prolactin, and growth hormone responses to handling and new environment in the rat. *Psychosom Med, 236*, 241.

Constantinou, J., & Korner, A. F. (1993). Neurobehavioral Assessment of the Preterm Infant as an instrument to enhance parental awareness. *Children's Health Care, 22*, 39–46.

Daily, W. J. R., Klaus, M., & Meyer, H. B. P. (1969). Apnea in premature infants: monitoring, incidence, heartrate changes, and an effect of environmental temperature [Part 1]. *J Pediatr, 43(4)*, 510–518.

Dreyfus-Brisac, C. (1974). Organization of sleep in prematures: implications for caretaking. In M. Lewis & L. A. Rosenblum (Eds.), *The Effect of the Infant on Its Caregiver*. New York: John Wiley.

Edelman, A. M., Kraemer, H. C., & Korner, A. F. (1982). Effects of compensatory movement stimulation on the sleep-wake behaviors of preterm infants. *J. Am Acad Child Psychia, 21(6)*, 555–559.

Erway, L. C. (1975). Otolith formation and trace elements: a theory of schizophrenic behavior. *J Orthomol Psychia, 4*, 16–26.

Goodlin, R. C. (1972). *Handbook of Obstetrical and Gynecological Data*. Los Altos, CA: Geron-X. p. 385.

Gottlieb, G. (1971). Ontogenesis of sensory function in birds and mammals. In E. Tobach, L. R. Aronson, & E. Shaw (Eds., (pp. 67–128). New York: Academic Press.

Gregg, C. L., Haffner, M. E., & Korner, A. F. (1976). The relative efficacy of vestibular-proprioceptive stimulation and the upright position in enhancing visual pursuit in neonates. *Child Dev, 47*, 309.

Harlow, H. (1958). The nature of love. *Am Psycho, 13*, 673–685.

Hofer, M. A. (1975). Infant separation responses and the maternal role. *Biol Psychia, 10(2),* 149–153.

Hofer, M. A. (1976). The organization of sleep and wakefulness after maternal separation in young rats. *Dev Psychobiol, 9(2),* 189–205.

Hooker, D. (1952). *The Prenatal Origin of Behavior.* Lawrence: University of Kansas Press.

Humphrey, T. (1965). The embryologic differentiation of the vestibular nuclei in man correlated with functional development. In *International Symposium on Vestibular and Oculomotor Problems.* Tokyo: Nippon-Hoeschst.

Infant Health and Development Program. (1990). Enhancing the outcomes of low-birthweight premature infants, a multi-site randomized trial. *JAMA, 263,* 3035–3042.

Jeannerod, M. (1969). Les mouvements du foetus pendant le sommeil de la mère. *Com Ren Soc Biol (Paris), 163(8/9),* 1843–1847.

Kleitman, N. (1969). Basic rest-activity cycle in relation to sleep and wakefulness. In A. Kales (Ed.), *Sleep Physiology and Pathology: A Symposium.* Philadelphia: J. B. Lippincott.

Korner, A. F. State as variable, as obstacle and as mediator of stimulation in infant research. *Merrill-Palmer Q, 18(2),* 77–94.

Korner, A. F. (1987). Preventive intervention with high-risk newborns: theoretical, conceptual and methodological perspectives. In J. D. Osofsky (Ed.), *Handbook for Infant Development* (2nd ed.). New York: Wiley-Interscience.

Korner, A. F. (1989). The scope and limitations of neurologic and behavioral assessments of the newborn. In D. K. Stevenson & P. Sunshine (Eds.), Fetal and Neonatal Brain Injury: Mechanisms, Management and the Risks of Practice (pp. 239–249). B. C, Decker.

Korner, A. F. (1996). Reliable individual differences in preterm infants' excitation management. *Child Dev, 67,* 1793–1805.

Korner, A. F., & Grobstein R. (1966). Visual alertness as related to soothing in neonates: implications for maternal stimulation and early deprivation. *Child Dev, 37(4),* 867–876.

Korner, A. F., & Thoman, E. B. (1970). Visual alertness in neonates as evoked by maternal care. *J Exp Child Psych, 10,* 67–78.

Korner, A. F., & Thoman, E. B. (1972). The relative efficacy of contact and vestibular stimulation in soothing neonates. *Child Dev, 43(2),* 443–453.

Korner, A. F., & Thom, V. A. (1990). Neurobehavioral Assessment of the preterm infant. The Psychological Corporation: San Antonio, TX.

Korner, A. F., Brown, Jr., B. W., Dimiceli, S., Forrest, T., Stevenson, D. K., Lane, N. M., Constantinou, J., & Thom V. A. Stable individual differences in developmentally changing preterm infants. *Child Dev, 60,* 502–513.

Korner, A. F., Brown, Jr, B. W., Reade, E. P., Stevenson, D. K., Fernback, S., & Thom, V. A. State behavior of preterm infants as a function of development, individual and sex differences. *Inf Behav Dev, 11,* 111–124.

Korner, A. F., Constantinou, J., Dimiceli, S., Brown, Jr, B. W., & Thom, V. A. (1991). Establishing the reliability and developmental validity of a neurobehavioral assessment for preterm infants: a methodological process. *Child Dev, 62(5),* 1200–1208.

Korner, A. F., Guilleminault, C., Van den Hoed, J., & Baldwin, R. C. (1978). Reduction of sleep apnea and bradycardia in preterm infants on oscillating waterbeds: a controlled polygraphic study. *Pediatrics, 61(4),* 528–533.

Korner A. F., Kraemer, H. C., Haffner M. E., & Cosper, L. M. (1975). Effects of waterbed flotation on premature infants: a pilot study. *Pediatrics, 56,* 361–367.

Korner, A. F., Kraemer, H. C., Reade, E. P., Forrest, T., Dimiceli, S., & Thom, V. A. A methodological approach to developing an assessment procedure for testing the neurobehavioral maturity of preterm infants. *Child Dev, 58,* 1478–1487.

Korner A. F., Ruppel E. M., & Rho, J. M. (1982). Effects of waterbeds on the sleep and motility of theophylline-treated preterm infants. *Pediatrics, 70,* 864–869.

Korner A. F., Schneider, P., & Forrest, T. (1983). Effects of vestibular-proprioceptive stimulation on the neurobehavioral development of preterm infants: a pilot study. *Neuropediatrics, 14(3),* 170–175.

Korner, A. F., Stevenson, D. K., Kraemer, H. C., Spiker, D., Scott, D. T., Constantinou, J., & Dimiceli, S. (1993). Prediction of the development of low-birthweight preterm infants by a new neonatal medical index. *J Dev Behav Ped, 14(2),* 106–111.

Korner, A. F., Stevenson, D. K., Forrest, T., Constantinou, J., Dimiceli, S., Brown, Jr, B. W. (1994). Preterm medical complications differentially affect neurobehavioral functions: results from a new neonatal medical index. *Inf Behav Dev,* 17, 37–43.

Langworthy, O. R. (1933). Development of behavior patterns and myelinization of the nervous system in human fetus and infant. *Contri Embryol, 24,* 1–57.

Lee, H. F. (1954). Rocking bed respirator for use with premature infants in incubators. *J Pediatr, 44,* 570–573.

Mason, W. A. (1968). Early social deprivation in the non-human primates: implications for human behavior. In D.C. Glass (Ed.), *Environmental Influences,* (p. 70). New York: Rockefeller University Press and Russell Sage Foundation.

Mason, W. A. (1979). Wanting and knowing: a biological perspective on maternal deprivation. In E. B. Thoman (Ed.), *Origins of the Infant's Social Responsiveness* (pp. 225–249). Hillsdale, NJ: Lawrence Erlbaum.

Millen R. S., & Davies, J. (1946). See-saw resuscitator for the treatment of asphyxia. *J. Obstet Gyn, 52,* 508–509.

Perlstein, P. H., Edwards, N. K., & Sutherland, J. N. (1970). Apnea in premature infants in incubator air temperature changes. *N Engl J Med, 282,* 461–466.

Saint-Anne Dagassies, S. (1966). Neurological maturation of the premature infant of 28 to 41 weeks' gestational age. In F. Falkner (Ed.), *Human Development* (pp. 306–325). Philadelphia Saunders.

Schanberg, S. M., Evoniuk, G., & Kuhn, C. M. (1984). Tactile and nutritional aspects of maternal care: specific regulators of neuroendocrine function and cellular development Proc *Soc Exp Biol Med,* 175–135–46.

Sterman, M. B. (1967). Relationship of intrauterine fetal activity to maternal sleep state. *Exp Neur Supp, 4,* 98–106.

Thoman, E. B., & Korner, A. F. (1971). Effects of vestibular stimulation on the behavior and development of infant rats. *Dev Psych, 5,* 92.

6

KANGAROO CARE OF THE PREMATURE INFANT

GENE CRANSTON ANDERSON

At birth, both full-term and preterm infants enter a foreign environment that lacks the skin-to-skin contact and close containment of extremities in the womb. This shock can be ameliorated by placing infants skin-to-skin with their mothers as soon as possible postbirth. When they are with their mothers, infants are in their ideal physiological and environmental milieu, that is, their ecological niche, which fosters a close dyadic relationship (Anderson, 1977). For preterm infants, however, the return to the mother may be delayed indefinitely.

Mother-infant separation following birth, with its sudden deprivation of maternal stimuli, has been the reason for numerous developmental interventions. Beginning in the 1960s, these interventions have been tested in full-term and preterm infants and have yielded useful and intriguing findings. A pressing questions for the 1990s is whether the delayed return of some preterm infants to the mother is always necessary or in their best interests.

Many parents express a strong need to hold their ill preterm infant, a fact well documented and understood. Perhaps parents sense that their infant needs to be held. Scientists must have sensed this need, as well, because several of the developmental interventions studied include holding techniques, for example, swaddling, carrying devices, containment, and full palmar massage. However, none of these interventions involves both skin-to-skin touching and full-body holding. Even full-term infants held in someone's arms were first capped and double-or triple-wrapped in blankets to preserve warmth. In spite of these precautions, preterm infants often became too cool. Fear of hypothermia is a major reason why neonatal intensive care unit (NICU) staffs have been reluctant to permit parents to hold their infants, especially very ill infants.

ADVENT OF KANGAROO CARE

This perspective began to change when Rey and Martinez (1983) from Bogotá, Colombia, reported dramatic success in decreasing mortality, morbidity, and infant abandonment by bringing mothers into their NICU. The mothers held their diaper-clad infants underneath their clothing, upright and skin-to-skin between their breasts, and allowed self-regulatory breastfeeding. Because this method resembles the way marsupials mother their young, it became known as *kangaroo care* (KC). Since then the method has been referred to as kangaroo baby care, kangaroo care, kangaroo method, kangaroo mother intervention, kangaroo mother method, mother kangaroo program, and skin-to-skin contact.[1] Rey and Martinez emphasized three important components: maternal warmth, maternal milk, and maternal love. News of favorable outcomes reached the United States in 1984 in communications from UNICEF. Disbelief was the almost unanimous response, which prompted UNICEF to investigate the research methods used.

Methodological flaws were indeed found by Whitelaw and Sleath (1985), who traveled to Bogotá. However, Whitelaw and Sleath were so impressed clinically by the KC they saw that, on their return to England, they began a systematic descriptive study of KC (Whitelaw, 1986), quickly followed by a randomized clinical trial (Whitelaw et al., 1988). Other researchers soon followed Whitelaw and Sleath to Bogotá, concurred with their conclusions, and documented that the infants were often appropriate in size for gestation and that KC did not begin until at least several hours postbirth (Anderson, Marks, & Wahlberg, 1986). These investigators were also impressed by what they saw clinically and began to study KC in the United States and Sweden.

Kangaroo care, as studied and implemented, fell into four general categories determined historically and based on a continuum of how soon KC began postbirth (Anderson, 1991). Regardless of category, complete KC includes self-regulatory breast-feeding, but this is not always possible. *Late kangaroo care* usually begins many days or weeks postbirth after the infant has completed the intensive care phase. *Intermediate kangaroo care* usually begins about 7 days after birth, while infants are still unstable (Figure 6.1) or stable on a ventilator. *Early kangaroo care* can begin during the first day, even the first few hours, for infants who can be stabilized prone in a warm incubator, with oxygen and intravenous fluids if necessary. *Very early kangaroo care* begins in the delivery or recovery room, usually between 30 and 40 minutes postbirth.

At two conferences in 1993, a 5th category was added, called *birth kangaroo care*, in which an infant is placed skin-to-skin on its mother's abdomen or in her arms during the first minute postbirth (Anderson, 1995). Birth KC for more

---

[1]In October 1996, leading researchers convened in Trieste, Italy, at a workshop organized and supported by the Bureau for International Health of the Instituto per l'Infanzia, which is a World Health Organization (WHO) Collaborating Centre for Maternal and Child Health (Bureau of International Health, 1996—Addendum). A more detailed report is in preparation. These researchers from around the world agreed to call the method *kangaroo mother care* (KMC) to achieve consistency. This term was not intended to exclude fathers but, rather, to focus on the centrality of the mother for her infant's care as well as the empowering she derives from this experience. However, the consensus statement derived from the workshop is presently in draft form and thus remains subject to change. Therefore, "kangaroo care," the term familiar to most of the potential readers of this text, is used throughout this chapter.

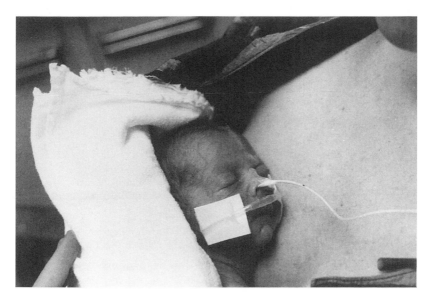

Figure 6.1. This is a 1250 gram, 29-week gestation infant who is appropriate for gestational age (AGA). He is now 7 days postbirth and is having his first KC on Mother's Day. This was also the first KC to occur at Children's Hospital of St. Paul, St. Paul, MN. This photograph is courtesy of the parents, Chris and Steve Clark, Cushing, WI, who learned about KC from an article in *Mothering* (Sims, 1988).

mature preterm infants was added to accommodate the method developed by Odent (1984, pp. 86–89), which Anderson described in more detail than is present in this chapter (1991, 1995). There are anecdotal reports from Sweden and Denmark; and published suggestions that birth KC may be the ideal intervention for larger preterm infants healthy at birth (Anderson, 1991, 1995; Bergman & Jürisoo, 1994; Davanzo, 1993).

RESEARCH FINDINGS

Earliest Research

Findings from most of the earlier research on KC (1986–1991) have been reviewed and organized by scientific rigor (Anderson, 1991), except for three publications identified later (Laine, 1987; Mondlane, de Graca, & Ebrahim, 1989; Wahlberg, 1991). Most of this research and descriptive work was done in Europe (Anderson, 1989b), although reports also came from Africa and North and South America. The findings, which were quite consistent across studies and a wide variety of research designs, permitted the general conclusion that KC was safe for most preterm infants and beneficial for some. Parents reaped benefits as well, becoming more attached, confident, and empowered.

During KC, preterm infants were warm enough; had adequate oxygenation; had less periodic breathing, apnea, and bradycardia; and had no increase in infection. Activity was reduced and behavioral state improved dramatically: almost no crying, twice as much deep sleep, longer episodes of deep sleep, and a 4-fold increase in alert inactivity. Infants tolerated room air sooner, went home sooner, and cried less at 6 months. With close observation, even very small, nonstabilized infants recently weaned from ventilators could tolerate KC, much to the benefit of their parents. These findings suggest a reduction in activity-and state-related energy expenditure (Anderson, 1991).

Mothers were more inclined to breast-feed, produced more milk, and breast-fed longer. Mothers felt close to their infants; became more comfortable about monitoring their infant's health, even in the NICU; and were not afraid to take their infants home. In one study, mothers who provided KC not only warmed their preterm infants effectively but demonstrated an amazing kind of "thermal synchrony"; their own body temperature increased or decreased as needed to maintain the temperatures of their infants in the thermoneutral range. Fathers also gave KC, and although not studied systematically, most father-infant responses were similar to those seen during maternal KC.

Recent Research

In general, the most recent research reports have larger samples than previous studies, more rigorous research designs, and dependent variables that are more often physiological and measured electronically. Data from these studies confirm earlier findings, provide some insight into mechanisms that may be operating during KC, and continue to suggest that KC is safe and effective.

Research Programs

The best example of this kind of research is an extensive research program in which a pulse oximeter, thermistor probes, and some form of cardiorespirograph are always used. Behavioral state and parental responses are studied as well. The first study was a pretest-test-posttest design with 12 preterm infants in open-air bassinets. The infants were studied on 1 day during 3 consecutive interfeeding intervals (Ludington-Hoe, Hadeed, & Anderson, 1991). Favorable responses on all dependent variables during KC permitted the conclusion that KC was safe for these infants and led to the second study with 24 similar infants and similar results. This study used the strongest kind of randomized clinical trial (RCT), with a pretest-test-posttest experimental control group design, and randomization was done with the Zelen technique. Thus, results are definitive. However, again KC was given only once (Ludington-Hoe et al., 1994).

This same design was next used with 41 incubator infants, some of whom had mild apnea and bradycardia (Ludington-Hoe & Swinth, 1994). These infants received intermediate KC. An advantage to this project was that KC was given over 5 consecutive days: for 3 hours on Days 1 and 5 and for at least 1 hour on Days 2, 3, and 4. Pretest-test-posttest measurements were done on Days 1 and 5. An ED-ENTECH four-channel real-time recorder was used, as well as a nasal airflow thermistor, to identify types of apnea (obstructive, central, or mixed) and their frequencies. No obstructive apnea occurred during KC. For Days 1 and 5 duration of apnea and apnea density (frequency and duration of apnea >6 seconds as percentage of quiet time) were determined. Both variables decreased from pretest to KC and increased from KC to posttest ($p < .001$), compared to no differences in the control infants. The authors concluded that KC was safe and effective in reducing the frequency and duration of apnea during KC. The current research tests the effects of KC in small, medically stable, ventilated preterm infants (Ludington, 1995–1997). A Gould physiograph is used for data collection (Ludington-Hoe & Kasper, 1995), and infants are randomized with an even more rigorous technique, the minimization method (Conlon & Anderson, 1990).

Another research program began in Helsingborg, Sweden (Wahlberg, 1991; Wahlberg, Affonso, & Persson, 1992). These investigators interviewed 33 healthy mothers, who gave early and intermediate KC in a secondary-level hospital. Their preterm infants were healthy and stable when first taken out of the incubator for KC. Thirty-three similar mothers in a retrospective control group were also interviewed. These mothers gave birth to similar infants, but gave no KC. The mothers were carefully matched between groups on seven potentially confounding variables: maternal age, parity, length of pregnancy, type of delivery, gestational age, birthweight, and technological intervention prior to first contact with mother outside the incubator. Maternal responses were compared and reported earlier (Affonso, Wahlberg, & Persson, 1989). Infants given KC were younger when they were first placed in open-air bassinets (4 days vs. 8), had greater weight gain per week (237 g vs. 196), had fewer days of incubator care (21 days vs. 30), had a shorter average length of hospital stay (42 days vs. 49), and were more frequently breast-fed upon discharge (82% vs. 45%).

Intermediate and late KC were studied next with eight mother-infant dyads in a tertiary care center in San Francisco, California (Bosque et al., 1995). All infants were cared for in incubators. Each mother gave KC a minimum of 4 hours each day for 6 days per week during a period of 3 consecutive weeks. Measurements before and during KC were similar for frequency and duration of apnea, bradycardia, heart rate, and oxygen saturation. During KC, compared to before, skin temperature was lower (36.5° vs. 36.8°C, $p < .03$) and percentage of sleep time was lower (47% vs. 64%, $p < .001$). However, these differences were not considered clinically important by the neonatology staff. A surprising finding emerged during the second week of KC, as each mother's emotions intensified and were manifested in fears for her infant's well-being, a need to discuss negative and positive emotional reactions to having a premature and sick baby, and a request for respite time from KC (Affonso et al., 1993b). Nevertheless, each mother emerged from this experience by the 3rd week with an increased sense of meaning, mastery, and self-esteem about having given birth to a preterm infant who required cardiovascular or respiratory assistance.

In Bogotá, Colombia, Charpak, Ruiz-Peláez, and Charpak (1994) were unable to do an RCT as a first step in their research program, but they did concurrently study two large cohorts of infants <2,000 grams: 162 infants at the kangaroo hospital, 170 at the control hospital. Kangaroo infants were discharged as soon as they became eligible for the Minimal Care Unit (MCU). Each mother was instructed to give the "full kangaroo intervention," which involved keeping her infant upright and in skin-to-skin contact on her chest 24 hours a day and providing self-regulatory breast-feeding. The KC infants came from a much lower socioeconomic class and were more ill before eligibility. In spite of these major baseline differences, survival was similar. However, the KC infants grew less the first 3 months and had more developmental delay at 1 year. Charpak et al. concluded that questions remain regarding quality of life, especially about weight gain and neurodevelopment, and that an RCT is needed. They are currently conducting an RCT at the former control hospital.

Components of KC

Specific components of KC are also being tested. For example, Legault and Goulet (1995) used a time-series repeated measures design with mother-infant dyads to compare KC holding and holding infants wrapped in blankets. The KC infants had less variation in oxygen saturation and tolerated KC for a longer time. And KC was preferred by most mothers.

In a methodological study, Sontheimer et al. (1995) found that during KC, infant respirations monitored with electrodes placed on the infant's chest did not record apneic pauses or sound the monitor's alarm because parental respirations were mistakenly recorded as infant respirations. However, bradycardia and oxygen saturation were recorded accurately at all times. Even with the electrodes placed on the infant's back, the problem persisted but to a much lesser degree. For this reason, and because Sontheimer et al. believe the advantages of KC far outweigh the disadvantages, they recommended that KC should continue, provided the electrodes are placed on the back and oxygen saturation and bradycardia are monitored.

Almost everyone eventually asks whether fathers can give KC to their infants. Ludington-Hoe et al. (1992) studied 11 healthy 34–36-week preterm infants given early KC by their fathers in Cali, Colombia. The KC was given for 2 hours beginning between 5 and 17 hours postbirth and immediately following a breast-feeding. Physiologic responses were recorded every minute. Infant heart rate, respiratory rate, and abdominal, toe, and core temperatures increased during KC. Abdominal temperature rose from an average of 36.4°C to 37.4°C (97.5°F to 99.3°F). Toe temperatures rose from 32.8°C to 35.3°C (91.0°F to 95.5°F). Toe temperature could be a valuable measure of condition, if it measures vasoconstriction (i.e., vascular perfusion) in infants as it does in adults. Infants slept most of the time while being held (65% of the time in quiet regular sleep and 7.5% in quiet irregular sleep), and fathers seldom gazed at, spoke to, or touched their infants while holding them. Despite cooling efforts, 5 infants became hyperthermic, perhaps due to the humid, warm environment (humidity 60% to 70%; 28.5°C to 32.0°C; 83.3°F to 89.6°F) and lack of air conditioning.

Published RCTs

To date, KC for preterm infants has been the intervention in only 2 published RCTs. In both trials the infants were given intermediate and late KC begun in the NICU when the infants were stable. The first RCT was done with 71 dyads in London, England, a developed country. The infants all weighed less than 1,500 grams when they were randomly assigned, on average 16 days postbirth. The KC dyads averaged 30 minutes of KC per day in hospital and were contacted again at 6 months. The KC mothers lactated 4 weeks longer, and KC infants cried 20 minutes less per day at 6 months (Whitelaw et al., 1988). The second RCT was done in Quito, Ecuador, a developing country, was planned for 700 dyads, and included a 6-month follow-up. The infants were <2,000 grams when they were randomly assigned, on average at 13 days postbirth. Sixty-eight percent of the sample were doing KC at 1 month, 47% at 1.5 months, 20% at 2 months, and 7% at 3 months. Mothers breast-fed in both groups. The trial was halted after 275 infants were studied, because the differences in severe morbidity (e.g., pneumonia) during the first 6 months were so significant (5% for KC infants, 18% for controls; p <.002). Mean overall costs were $741 greater for control infants. The KC mothers made more unscheduled visits for their infants, other children, and themselves than control mothers, but KC infants had fewer readmissions so the cost of care was lower. Control mothers made fewer clinic visits for themselves but had almost twice as many multiple illnesses prompting these visits, suggesting higher maternal morbidity.

Kangaroo Care for Ventilated Infants

The first report of KC given to infants receiving mechanical ventilation came from Norway (Gloppestad, 1987). Compared to a historical control group, the separation time before fathers were first allowed to hold their ventilated infants in KC was reduced by 67% (Gloppestad, 1995). Gale et al. (1993) studied 25 intubated preterm infants given late KC by their mothers ($n = 24$) and fathers ($n = 7$). All infants had respiratory distress syndrome and were at risk for bronchopulmonary dysplasia; 24% had mothers who abused cocaine prenatally. Gale et al. concluded that their method was safe and promoted parental attachment, even in parents at high risk for impaired attachment. It should be noted, however, that their method included the assistance of a neonatal development nurse, who was experienced in infant development and tertiary neonatal nursing and who stayed with the parents. This nurse's presence was reported as being reassuring to both the parents and the NICU nurses.

Currently, KC is being done with intubated infants at dozens of sites, because anecdotal reports from clinical practice have been so favorable (e.g., Drosten-Brooks, 1993; Gale et al., 1993; Gloppestad, 1987; Wallace & Ridpath-Parker, 1993). However, a controversy still exists about the advisability of this practice. In fact, de Leeuw (de Leeuw et al., 1991; de Leeuw, 1992) advised against it and Ludington-Hoe, Thompson, et al. (1994) agree, reasoning that no RCTs had been done to determine the safety and effectiveness of this intervention (see also Ludington-Hoe, Anderson, et al., 1994). Gale et al. recommended caution in adapting their method to other NICUs and called for prospective investigation to determine the effectiveness of KC for intubated infants as compared to standard care. As mentioned previously, an RCT with small, medically stable, intubated infants is in progress (Ludington, 1995–1997).

Very Early KC

As clinicians and investigators become more familiar with KC, they are beginning to offer it sooner postbirth, not just with sicker and smaller infants, but
also with the healthiest preterm infants, who have the best chance for normal
development and who may not need to be in the NICU at all. In another
research program, KC beginning in the delivery room has been studied in 3
projects with infants who are healthy at birth, who are 34–36 weeks gestation,
and whose mothers have chosen to breast-feed. The objective here is to see if
this close and continuous skin-to-skin contact with the mother and self-regulatory
feeding will help to maintain the health of these infants, thereby eliminating the
need for admission to the NICU.

In the first project, six infants were studied descriptively in Cali, Colombia.
All had KC, on average, from 26 minutes to 6.5 hours postbirth. Two infants
(34 and 36 weeks gestation) developed grunting respirations by the time KC
began, but the grunting resolved quickly with continued KC and warmed humidified oxygen via oxyhood (Figure 6.2). The nurse researchers stayed with
each mother-infant dyad during the first 6.5 hours postbirth. Then the infants

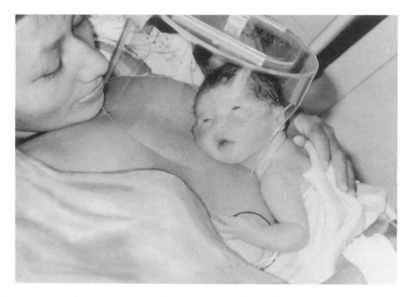

Figure 6.2. This is a 34-week gestation infant from Cali, Colombia, who
weighs 2160 grams and is AGA. She began grunting just as she started
KC about 19 minutes postbirth. She was given warmed and humidified
oxygen via oxyhood and the grunting disappeared within 8 minutes. She
is shown here at 90 minutes postbirth just before the oxyhood was removed. Her Dextrostix was 90 mg% at 2 ¾ hours postbirth. KC continued
until 6 hours postbirth, when she and her mother were transferred to
the postpartum ward. She was fully breastfeeding and approved for
discharge the next day (Ludington et al., 1993). (Photograph by this author)

went to the postpartum ward with their mothers; they were fully breast-feeding and ready for discharge 24–36 hours postbirth (Ludington-Hoe et al., 1993). In the second project, 14 similar Colombian infants, all grunting, were given very early KC with similar results. The first 6 infants in this series have been reported (Argote et al., 1991).

The third project was a pilot RCT conducted with infants in the United States (Syfrett et al., 1993a, 1993b). Eight infants were randomly assigned at 1 hour postbirth to the KC group or the hospital routine-care group. Three infants developed grunting during the first hour postbirth. After random assignment, 2 of these infants were in the KC group and 1 in the control group. The nurse researchers stayed with the KC dyads and supported each mother by helping her to breast-feed, keep her infant warm, and recognize her infant's cues and respond to them appropriately. Fathers became involved, also (Figure 6.3). All infants thermoregulated rapidly, showed outstanding behavioral organization, became competent breast-feeders by 24 hours postbirth, received no supplementation, and were discharged in 3.8 days, on average. They stayed with their mothers until their mothers were discharged; then they were cared for in the normal newborn nursery. Their mothers rapidly developed a large milk volume, had no signs of engorgement, and had no complaints of breast or nipple pain. The control infants were discharged in 14.2 days on average, spending 3 days in the NICU and 5.8 days in the stepdown unit. At 1-year follow-up, breast-

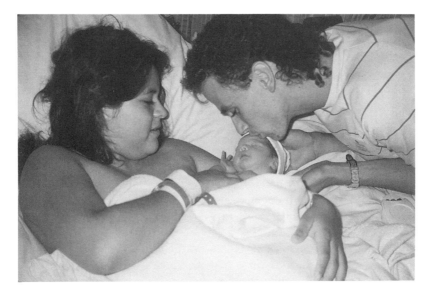

Figure 6.3. This is a 2480 gram, 34-week gestation infant who is AGA. His 16-year-old mother was induced for severe preeclampsia at Shands Hospital at the University of Florida, Gainesville, FL. He is shown here with his parents at 16 hours postbirth. He is already a competent breast-feeder (Syfrett et al., 1993a, 1993b). (Photograph by this author)

feeding duration was shorter for the control infants (1.5 months vs. 3.7), and their morbidity was more severe on all comparisons. This pilot work has led to an RCT in progress with 100 mothers whose infants are 32–35 weeks gestation, weigh 1,500 to < 2,500 grams, are singletons born vaginally or by cesarean section, and are breast-fed or bottle-fed. The infants are randomly assigned at 10 minutes postbirth. Follow-up will be done for 18 months (Anderson et al., 1996–2000).

Birth KC

Johanson et al. (1992) studied 300 infants in an RCT in Kathmandu, Nepal, to determine the effect of postdelivery care on neonatal body temperature. Approximately 22% of the infants weighed < 2,500 grams; half of these infants were small for gestation but not preterm, and half were preterm. At birth the infants were dried off and randomized to a warm mustard oil massage and radiant heater group, a plastic wrap and blanket-swaddled group, or a birth KC group. Mean air temperatures were 20.0°C (68.0°F) at 2 hours and 17.8°C (64.0°F) at 24 hours. Although direct correlations were found between gestation and temperature, data for preterm and low birthweight (LBW) full-term infants were not reported separately, so no conclusions can be drawn for preterm infants alone.

Johanson et al. concluded that all 3 interventions were equally effective at 2 and 24 hours postbirth, provided the infants were dried well immediately after birth. However, at 2 and 24 hours postbirth, numerous KC infants had temperatures < 36°C (< 96.8°F) and some < 35°C (< 95°F), a highly unusual finding compared to similar studies of KC. One explanation at 2 hours might lie in the following comment by the authors: "If the clothing was considered insufficient, the baby was swaddled in one of the labour room blankets and then kept immediately against the mother." This is no longer KC. Even a single layer of a thin receiving blanket between the mother and her infant can compromise the warming process during this early time postbirth (Syfrett et al., 1993b). It is also important for the just-delivered infant to wear a cap and, if it becomes damp, to replace it with a dry cap. At 24 hours the explanation might be that the mothers were not sufficiently convinced about the importance of keeping their infant skin-to-skin and were not being carefully monitored.

Birth KC has been studied also as it was being implemented. Upon arrival at the Manama Mission Hospital in Manama, Zimbabwe, Bergman and Jürisoo (1994) found that the hospital was poorly equipped, for example, totally without incubators, and the survival rate of LBW infants (LBWIs) was very low. They decided to implement KC exclusively for *all* infants born at or admitted to the hospital, and they began KC for 133 consecutive LBWIs "within minutes of delivery." This avoided methodological problems in earlier studies using historical control groups (Martinez, Rey, & Marquette, 1992) and permitted valid comparison with a historical control group drawn before the introduction of KC. Survival improved from 10% to 50% for infants < 1,500 grams and from 70% to 90% for infants 1,500–1,999 grams. Bergman and Jürisoo concluded that stabilization and subsequent care of LBW newborns were achieved by using KC.

Ironically, a very similar approach, although with more selective admission, became routine practice in 1979 at the Cambridge Maternity Hospital in Cambridge, England. Whitby, de Cates, and Roberton (1982) designated 1 of their 4 postnatal wards to accept asymptomatic infants weighing 1,800 to 2,500 grams, including twins, higher multiples, and infants with malformations whose lives were not threatened. These infants were admitted directly from the labor ward and were cot-nursed and roomed in with their mothers just like the normal birthweight infants on the ward. Whitby et al. reported detailed outcomes for a 13-month period with 269 consecutive infants who met the above inclusion criteria. They concluded that the program was highly successful. The ward was easy to run and popular with nursing staff and mothers. Thus, 19 years ago this kind of care was documented as possible and valuable in a developed country.

Since the research by Whitby et al. (1982), other leaders in the field have endorsed a similar approach. Fourteen years ago, Kennell and Klaus recommended that "the focus should be on this large group of more mature premature infants who may inadvertently be separated and exposed to conditions that could, over a period of time, be detrimental to their developmental needs" (1985, p. 273). Davanzo made the following statement in the guidelines he prepared for WHO after 4 years of working in Mozambique, where KC was provided beginning several days postbirth: "As a matter of fact, we do not know if it is really safer for LBWIs in developing countries to remain initially in the incubator instead of entering immediately the K-M (Kangaroo-Mother) method. Well designed randomized studies should investigate this important aspect" (1993, p. 14).

Research has also been done with full-term infants given birth KC (Christensson et al., 1992; Curry, 1982; Färdig, 1980; Righard & Alade, 1990; Righard & Frantz, 1992; Widström et al., 1987; Widström, Ransjö-Arvidson, & Christensson, 1993). A discussion of this research is beyond the scope of this chapter, except to say that full-term infants clearly benefit from birth KC and very early KC.

WHY IS KANGAROO CARE EFFECTIVE?

Numerous mechanisms can be offered to explain the effectiveness of kangaroo (skin-to-skin) care. Conceivably more than one could be operating, concurrently or sequentially. One mechanism alluded to earlier is the continuity hypothesis. Simply stated, certain stimuli become salient to the fetus and, if presented to the infant after birth, will have soothing and regulating effects (Ourth & Brown (1961). The mother provides the optimal familiar milieu for her infant. She and her infant function as partners as they interact together in a self-regulatory way. Part of the idea of self-regulation is that newborn infants are able to tell us what they need by giving cues. They do not need to cry to communicate stress if we are willing to watch them patiently, learn to recognize when they are giving cues, and read and respond to these cues appropriately (Gill, White, & Anderson, 1984).

Crisis theory (Rapaport, 1965, p. 25) and stress theory provide another mechanism. Birth, followed by separation from the mother, meets the definition of a crisis for the infant. Infants cry significantly more when separated after birth (Anderson, 1989a) and cease to cry when reunited (Christensson et al., 1995). In an RCT with 84 full-term infants, salivary (unbound) cortisol was significantly higher at 6 hours postbirth in the infants separated from their mothers, compared to those who stayed with their mothers (9.1 ng/ml vs. 4.1 ng/ml, $p <$ .05) (Anderson et al., 1995). This finding suggests that separation during these early hours after birth was stressful for these infants. The lower cortisol in the KC infants may explain the stress-free expression that infants typically assume during KC (Anderson, 1995; Figure 6.4). Physiologically, cortisol is an accepted index of stress, and salivary cortisol is a highly accurate index of the tissue fraction, for example, in the brain. Elevated cortisol as the result of maternal-infant separation in the early postbirth period has life-span adverse effects on responsivity to stress, at least in the rat model (see review by Meaney et al., 1994, pp. 252–256).

Another explanation for the effectiveness of KC takes into consideration that the transitional newborn infant is uniquely vulnerable during the intrauterine-extrauterine adaptation, the greatest physiological adaptation ever required of the human organism. I suggest this adaptation is delayed and sometimes compromised by crying (1989a). Crying is a modified Valsalva maneuver and the epitomy of irregular respiration. The prolonged expiration (strain phase) of the cry raises intrathoracic pressure, so that pulmonary pressure is higher than systemic pressure, thereby reversing the ideal pressure relationship established when the lungs expand at birth. Venous return to the heart is also obstructed during the strain phase. When the strain is released, as much as $^2/_3$ of the poorly oxygenated blood coming into the heart forces its way through the foramen ovale and into the systemic circulation, introducing some degree of hypoxemia (Lind, Stern, & Wegelius, 1964/1974). Thus portions of the fetal circulatory pattern are reestablished. With regular respirations, the opposite is true: venous return is modulated and the blood returning to the heart flows to the lungs and becomes reoxygenated; this should facilitate physiologic (functional) closure first and then closure of the foramen ovale and the ductus arteriosus (Anderson, 1989a). During KC the respirations become remarkably regular, and crying rarely occurs (Anderson, 1995; Ludington-Hoe, Thompson, et al., 1994).

Uvnäs-Moberg et al. (1987) found that activation of sensory nerves in the oral mucosa, nipple, or skin leads to an activation of vagally mediated hormone secretion from the gut and the pituitary. They conclude that many types of neurogenic reflexes induced in mother-infant interactions are important for the energy economy of the mother and her infant. These effects are also seen when nonnutritive sucking is provided during tube feedings (Widström et al., 1988). These data support earlier research in which 2 newly delivered moribund lambs with respiratory distress sucked eagerly on the investigator's finger and recovered

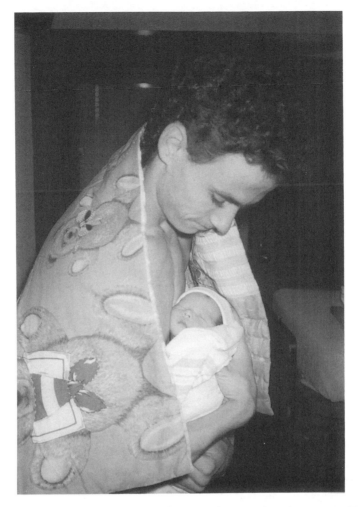

Figure 6.4. This is the same infant as the one in Figure 6-3. Here his father is giving KC for the first time at about 10 hours postbirth. The peaceful relaxed expression on the infant's face is very common during KC (Syfrett et al., 1993a, 1993b). (Photograph by this author)

almost immediately. These events led to the hypothesis that nonnutritive sucking, via vagal stimulation, releases surfactant from glandular elements in the epithelial lining of the pulmonary alveoli (Anderson, 1975). The fact that the epithelial lining of the lungs buds from the embryologic gut, and thus is similar in structure, lends credence to this hypothesis. Also supportive are similar findings with human infants (Argote et al., 1991; Van Art & Higgins, 1977) and the fact that, in contrast to crying, respirations are remarkably regular during nonnutritive sucking (Wolff, 1966), just as they are during KC.

Because infants are asleep between 50% and 75% of the time during KC (Ludington-Hoe, 1990; Ludington-Hoe, Thompson, et al., 1994), KC can be considered a form of co-sleeping. McKenna reported that he and his colleague, Sarah Mosko, found that co-sleeping mothers and infants exhibited synchronous, partner-induced physiological arousals. They also found that co-sleeping infants spent less time in deep stages of sleep and more in higher stages than infants sleeping alone. They propose that solitary sleep environments may accelerate the maturation of deep sleep, possibly before arousal mechanisms are maximally efficient to achieve arousals during some physiological crises. They further propose that co-sleeping gives the young infant practice in arousal, and this practice may be needed in order to balance the tendency to fall into deep sleep from which some infants may have difficulty arousing (McKenna et al., 1993). Perhaps this perspective is relevant to the 4-fold decrease in apnea and bradycardia found in preterm infants during KC (Ludington & Swinth, 1994).

Five other mechanisms will be mentioned briefly. First, an energy conservation mechanism is justified by findings of improved behavioral state (Ludington-Hoe, 1990). Second, KC appears to increase a mother's desire and her ability to breast-feed, which increases the likelihood that KC infants will receive the many benefits of species-specific, gestation-specific, and antibody-specific breast milk. The last three mechanisms are most specific to very early KC and birth KC: colostrum becomes available to the infant during the first hour or two, which may be when it can be most beneficial; any circadian rhythms established with the mother while in utero would probably be preserved; and, because the newly delivered infant stays warm during KC, as reported by Syfrett et al. (1993a, 1993b), complications of hypothermia can be avoided.

STATUS QUO OF KANGAROO CARE

Kangaroo care has become virtually standard policy in Scandinavia, is proliferating across Africa, the United States, and Western Europe, and has begun in Canada (Hamelin & Ramachandran, 1993; Legault & Goulet, 1995), Eastern Europe (Levin, 1994), India, and the Pacific Rim. Breast-feeding is an integral part of KC in most nations but is seen as only optimal in the United States, where it is much less common. Wide variation in use of KC exists in the United States, ranging from complete implementation to complete resistance. To date, parents tend to acquiesce when KC is not allowed. Nevertheless, numerous recent developments indicate considerable progress.

Recent Developments

Increasing awareness of and interest in KC is evident among health professionals, lay persons, and the media in the United States. A paperback on KC (Ludington-Hoe & Golant, 1993) is partly responsible, as well as reports in the media, for example, *Baby Talk, Good Morning America, Ladies' Home Journal, Mothering, New York Times, Prevention,* and *Reader's Digest.* In the latest edition of his widely read book, Nilsson (1990, pp. 170–171, 180) included photographs of a father giving KC to his very weak infant and a mother holding her infant to her breast during gavage feeding.

Word about KC also spreads when it is implemented in a tertiary referral center, because information can be shared with staff from referring hospitals through outreach educational programs (Drosten-Brooks, 1993; Victor & Persoon, 1994). Often a care plan for KC is sent along when an infant is transferred back to the referring hospital. This anticipatory guidance not only aids parents who want to continue KC but introduces the concept very specifically to another hospital. Soon a cluster of KC hospitals develops. Bergman and Jürisoo (1994) extended this idea to in-transfers, as well, teaching KC to the rural hospitals near Manama, Zimbabwe, so that referred infants will arrive warm.

A survey of NICUs in the United States brought responses from 99 units in which KC was being practiced. Fifty of these units were giving KC to intubated infants. The survey was done in part to develop a list of NICUs willing to serve as resource units. This list is available from Gay Gale, BSN, Children's Hospital, Oakland Child Development Center, 747 52nd Street, Oakland, California 94609.

Aside from helping the surviving infant, KC can be helpful for newborn infants with a fatal anomaly. Collins (1993) presents a case study about a newborn infant with renal agenesis and resultant pulmonary hypoplasia, circumstances incompatible with life. The infant was given supportive care, including mechanical ventilation. The mother, who had a cesarean section, was brought to the NICU in her hospital bed. The baby, Stephanie, lived for 17 hours during which she was given KC, her vital signs remained stable, and she required no sedation. Her peacefulness convinced family and staff alike that, under the circumstances, she had been provided with an optimal environment for the dying process, which also allowed both bonding and grieving to take place for the family.

Similarly, KC can be helpful when an infant's condition worsens and the decision is made to remove the ventilatory support because further treatment would be futile. At this time the infant can be given to the parents to hold in KC. In fact, two anecdotal reports are circulating about infants like this, who began to improve after KC began and ultimately survived. In one case, this event precipitated the ongoing use of KC in that NICU.

The forerunner of conferences on KC was a WHO Consensus Conference held in Trieste, Italy. The general topic was simple and appropriate technologies for the care of LBWIs, with strong emphasis placed on KC (WHO, 1985). Since then, 3 international conferences concerning KC have been held: the first in Bogotá, Colombia, sponsored by the UNICEF Regional Office for Latin America and the Caribbean (Martinez & Aguilar, 1992) in 1990 and the second in Boston, Massachusetts (Brigham & Women's Hospital, 1993). The third conference was the workshop mentioned in footnote 1 (Bureau of International Health, 1996). One purpose was to present and discuss the results of a multicenter study of KC in 5 developing countries: Brazil, Ethiopia, India, Indonesia, and Mexico. The study was supported by the study sites, the Bureau of International Health in Trieste, and WHO. Two other purposes were for the other KC researchers to present their results for discussion and for the entire group to reach a consensus on the indications and requirements for KC in three model settings (see the Addendum to the report).

The concept of *kangaroo care* has gained acceptance. The first evidence of this was inclusion of "kangaroo care" in the Word Watch section of *The Atlantic* (Soukhanov, 1992, p. 127). A nurse theorist has discussed KC in relation to her theory of energy conservation (Levine, 1991). And KC has been acknowledged in other ways. Leaders in the International Childbirth Educators Association (ICEA) now recommend that information about KC be added to their prenatal curriculum, so that parents are informed of this option in advance of need. In one hospital a preceptorship has been established for staff nurses who want to learn about KC (Drosten-Brooks, 1993). In 2 separate instances, KC has been incorporated into hospital policy as well: in one hospital, KC is included as a competency that nurses must pass to work in a NICU; in another hospital, an incident report must be filed whenever parents are not informed about KC. In addition, KC has been classified as a nursing intervention (McCloskey & Bulechek, 1995).

Current Guidelines

General guidelines for KC are as follows. Before coming to the hospital, KC caregivers should take a shower or wash their chest area and wear a clean V-neck top that is somewhat stretchy or a shirt, blouse, or dress that buttons or zips at least to the waist. When they arrive at the hospital, they may wish to wear a long-sleeved hospital gown backwards so that it opens down the front. The gown can be worn either over the caregiver's clothing, or the blouse or shirt can be removed. In either case, women should remove their brassiere to increase comfort and amount of skin-to-skin contact. Infants should wear only a small diaper. If their temperature is low, they should never be wrapped in a blanket; instead, a blanket can be placed over the infant's back, or a large blanket can be placed over the infant and the caregiver. If the amount of time the caregiver can stay is limited, it is best to arrive about 1 hour before a scheduled feeding and try to stay through the next feeding. The caregivers need to be gentle, relaxed, and reasonably quiet. Being gentle promotes relaxation for them as well as for the infant.

For more detailed guidelines see Davanzo (1993), de Leeuw (1986), Drosten-Brooks (1993), Gale et al. (1993), Levin (1994), Ludington, Thompson et al. (1994), Martinez et al. (1992), and Moeller-Jensen et al. (1987). Useful guidelines for birth KC are presented by Bergman & Jürisoo (1994) and Whitby et al. (1982). Between KC sessions, ongoing developmental care (Als et al., 1986; Als et al., 1994) is probably the best alternative.

Typically, KC begins by transferring the infant to the parent who is sitting in a chair. A new technique, the "standing transfer," may be easier on the infant, however. The parent stands next to the incubator so that the nurse can transfer the infant directly to the parent; thus, the infant is not suspended in and moved through midair. The nurse then guides the parent and the monitoring and intravenous lines to the chair. The standing transfer can also be done with the parents placing their hands under their infants and lifting them to their chests themselves. Some investigators have recommended that 2 nurses assist in transferring intubated infants (Drosten-Brooks, 1993), but others feel that 1 experienced nurse can do the transfer alone (Gale et al., 1993).

Of course, KC can be given in a brisk and seemingly efficient manner by nurses or parents, but "taking time" and "being gentle" are essential to KC's optimal effectiveness. Pickler (1993), who studied preterm infants at 24 to 26 weeks gestation ($M = 29$), documented their cues and different nurse caregiver styles in terms of initiating care (do the nurses alert or precipitate?), transacting during care (do they pace set or just do the task?), and concluding care (do they wind down or withdraw?). She found that infant physiologic and behavioral responses were dramatically more positive to the alerting, pace setting, and winding down caregiver style, which is similar to maternal handling. Unless maternal handling interfered with the infant's rest, Murdoch and Darlow (1984) found that it had a benign effect on transcutaneous arterial oxygen monitoring, compared to handling for procedures.

Drosten-Brooks (1993) recommends that all infants be gently awakened before transfer into KC and that all transfers occur in a dimly lit, quiet, rather private environment, where everyone involved speaks in whispers. Especially at first, or if the infant is quite ill, parents are asked to speak softly and briefly to their infant and not to rock the chair, lest the infant become overstimulated. Perhaps KC could begin earlier if done consistently, using the standing transfer and the caregiver styles just described.

BRINGING KANGAROO CARE INTO THE NICU

An important first step in promoting KC is to become thoroughly knowledgeable about the method. The following process is recommended. Write to me for a packet of selected research articles, reviews, guidelines, current bibliography, and list of recommended speakers. Make copies for your staff. Hold group discussions and address concerns raised. Then have an inservice and demonstration by someone who has already implemented KC. Offer to start with the strongest infants and the most eager and responsible parents. Offer to monitor and strip-record the infant's physiologic responses before, during, and after KC. Also follow their daily weights. The KC packet contains 4 legal forms available for parents to sign, if a physician is reluctant to permit KC for fear a malpractice suit might result. The 4 forms are designed for use by parents in the following circumstances: when the mother is in preterm labor, after a preterm infant has been born, for a preterm infant who has developed bronchopulmonary dysplasia, and for a preterm infant who may have been cocaine-exposed *in utero*.

If unsuccessful at this point, remember that those hospital staff who are resistant to KC vary in what touches them. Some staff only value KC as a means of promoting attachment or mother's milk supply. However, KC can also have a positive effect on the infant's physiologic function. Thus, it is important to identify the staff concerns and take the opportunity to introduce KC at the right time. If an infant is restless and not gaining weight, KC can be suggested (Anderson, 1995). If an infant is having apnea and bradycardia, suggest that these episodes may decrease, at least during the time KC is being given (Ludington-Hoe & Swinth, 1994; Ludington-Hoe, Thompson, et al., 1994). Sometimes nurses who are reluctant to use KC can be reached best by a father wanting to do KC. Also, KC can be suggested if there is concern on the unit about parents who show little interest in their infant. One KC experience is often all it takes to turn this lack of interest around, both for parents and for resistant staff. From a different perspective, neonatologists in one suburban setting have become very supportive of KC because of numerous spontaneous monetary contributions from satisfied families. Increased parental satisfaction has potential for increased market share (Wallace & Ridpath-Parker, 1993).

If the physicians in the unit value mothers providing breast milk, suggest KC when a mother is having difficulty letting down to the breast pump or is beginning to lose her milk supply. For infants who are too weak to breast-feed, suggest KC with the infant at the mother's breast during tube feedings. If this is done frequently, infants can go directly from tube feeding to breast-feeding. Even complete feeding by cup is possible (Armstrong & Kamau, 1986; Bergman & Jürisoo, 1994; IBFAN, 1990; Lang, Lawrence, & Orme, 1994). In research by Meier (1988), preterm infants who were beginning oral feedings had more stable and higher $tcPO_2$, were warmer, and had no apnea or bradycardia during breast-feeding compared to bottle-feeding.

Parents can become interested in KC in many ways. If mothers seem uninterested, perhaps even apathetic or depressed, they usually respond very positively when they try KC. Thus, some encouragement by staff and other parents can be justified. The video by Rosenberg and Balmes (1995) is a helpful adjunct.

An additional incentive for parents may be that frequent KC is likely to help their baby's head stay nicely rounded (Figure 6.5) (Chan, Kelley, & Khan, 1993; Schwirian, Eesley, & Cuellar, 1986). The skulls of preterm infants are particularly vulnerable to deformity (Peabody & Lewis, 1985), because stiffness of fetal skull bone increases up to 10-fold in the last 10 weeks of gestation and is highly correlated with birthweight (Kriewall, 1982). Baum and Searls (1971) found that deformity persists into adulthood. All anecdotal reports indicate that KC minimizes bilateral head flattening, though prospective research remains to be done. Methods of measuring head flattening have been reported by Chan et al. and Schwirian et al.

And KC has begun in other ways. For example, an article about KC in a popular magazine (Sims, 1988) resulted in requests by a mother and father in 1 NICU (Victor & Persoon, 1994) and a group of parents in another. Elsewhere, a mother who had not been allowed to hold or breast-feed her infant began threatening to disconnect the baby from all her tubes and wires and take her home. In all these cases, the staff was familiar with KC but had not yet tried it.

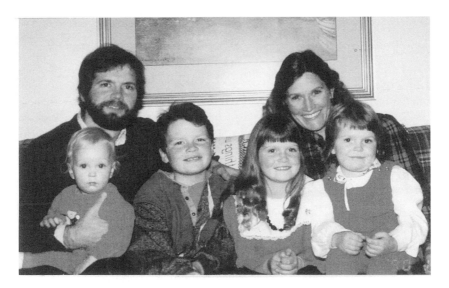

Figure 6.5. Here the infant seen in Figure 6.1 is 1½ years of age. Note the well-shaped head with no indication of cranial deformity from mattress pressure. The KC time increased from two 30-minute sessions per day to two 2–3-hour sessions over a 54-day period. (Photograph cortesy of parents)

Implementation

Implementing a program of KC is qualitatively different from having an occasional parent or parents give KC. With implementation, all parents are informed about KC and its safety and possible benefits, they are encouraged to try KC when their infant is ready, and they are promised assistance. Victor and Persoon (1994) described how this process was carried out at St. Paul Children's Hospital in St. Paul, Minnesota the first NICU to fully implement KC in the United States. Wallace and Ridpath-Parker (1993) described the process of involving and supporting staff and parents as KC was implemented at Brigham & Women's Hospital in Boston. Key steps for staff included developing a brochure, protocols, and guidelines and meeting regularly to give one another feedback and support. Key steps for parents included holding weekly meetings, creating a family advisory board, and distributing parent satisfaction questionnaires. Questionnaire results were shared with staff with the expectation that staff would be accountable to the parents for expressed concerns.

Facilitation

The original KC model, which represents the ideal, was observed in 1988 at Helsingborg Hospital in Helsingborg, Sweden (Anderson, 1989b). This comprehensive model was so successful that all major hospitals in Sweden sent hospital staff to Helsingborg to learn the method. Helsingborg Hospital is a secondary-level hospital, but much that has been developed there for KC can be adapted to a tertiary care NICU, such as the Infant Development Unit and Program described by Graven (1983).

Respect and convenience for families are major goals at Helsingborg, along with creating a family-friendly, "homey" environment. The unit is cheerful, neat, clean, and decorated in bright colors and with touches of humor. A private place is provided for parents to change and store clothes. A small but attractive kitchen has a table and 4 chairs, a microwave oven, and a refrigerator stocked with fruit juice and yogurt. Families can bring food from home to store and heat later. The unit also has a play corner for siblings, a telephone just for families to use, and couches, television, a baby buggy, and comfortable reclining chairs. Very small rooms with beds are provided so mothers can stay overnight with their infants, especially when the infant is ready to fully breast-feed and also shortly before discharge. These units are part of the breast-feeding model developed by Berlith Persson and described in greater detail by Wahlberg (1991). Moeller-Jensen et al. (1987) report that telemetry has been used for years in Sønderborg, Denmark, so that the infant can be evaluated without a direct connection to the monitors. This means that the parents are able to walk about the larger unit while doing KC.

Perhaps most important, facilitation of KC at Helsingborg involves having 1 contact nurse for each infant and family. This nurse meets with the family to individualize the care plan as much as necessary to meet that family's particular needs. Needs vary between families and also tend to change within families over time. Therefore, care plans are frequently reevaluated.

Limitations of KC

For all its effectiveness, KC does have some limitations. The need for gentle handling and low-level stimulation has already been discussed, as has the fact that infants can get too warm, especially with fathers in a warm environment. Infants who are too warm should have their head, hands, and feet uncovered. The extremities are very temperature-sensitive and exposing them will help cool the infant. Conversely, head, hands, and feet must be covered when trying to warm an infant, and ventral skin-to-skin contact must be preserved. Thus, the infant must not be wrapped. Instead a blanket can be placed over the infant's back. The KC caregiver needs to be kept warm as well, but any covering must be placed over the backs of the mother and infant, not between them.

Although obstructive apnea has not been reported during KC, Ludington-Hoe, Thompson, et al. (1994) warn that it could occur in the KC position. Thus, the nurse must remain vigilant and caution parents that smaller, younger, and sicker incubator-care infants have less mature muscle tone and need some assistance to keep from slouching. Reclining chairs help maintain optimal infant position. Infants may also assume a very flexed position at first, but there is a solution for this. After 2 or 3 minutes, flexed infants will begin to relax and then can be gently massaged to a stretched-out position, which helps them relax and also increases the area of ventral skin-to-skin contact.

Direct comparisons of KC with and without breast-feeding have not been made, so nothing definitive can be said regarding whether breast-feeding enhances KC and its effects. Nevertheless, mothers who choose to breast-feed or to provide expressed breast milk benefit from a supportive and well-informed NICU staff. Although thorough discussion of this topic is beyond the scope of this chapter, the following references are offered for interested readers: Armstrong & Kamau (1986), Bergman & Jürisoo (1994), Kyenkya-Isabirye (1992), Lang et al., (1994), Lawrence (1994), Meier (1988), Meier et al., (1993), Riordan & Auerbach (1993), and U.S. Department of Health and Human Services, Division of Maternal and Child Health (1985). Meier et al. provide an ideal introduction and the most specific information.

Affonso et al. (1993a) documented the consistent phenomenon of maternal emotional crisis in their San Francisco sample of 8 mothers of high-risk infants in the NICU. The mothers had agreed to give KC for at least 4 hours 6 days a week for 3 consecutive weeks. However, sometime during the 2nd week each mother expressed feelings of fatigue and stress and asked to be excused from KC for an extra day. All the mothers then resumed daily KC until the end of the study. This experience of emotional crisis may seem a limitation, but instead it probably represents a necessary growth step for the mother, resulting from increasing feelings of love for her infant and leading to her acceptance of the reality of the preterm birth and its risks, as well as the responsibility she must assume for her infant (Affonso et al., 1993a; Anderson, 1993). The development of healthy attachment can then follow. Awareness that this phenomenon can occur will alert NICU staff to beginning symptoms, so that additional support can be provided at this time. A question not yet answered is whether the mother can be helped, through anticipatory guidance, by explaining what may happen or has begun to happen to her and that many women experience this, or whether she needs to work through the entire experience on her own in order to achieve optimal benefit. Another question is whether this phenomenon occurs in all mothers who give KC to their ill preterm infants or just in certain subgroups.

Another limitation is the labor-intensive nature of KC for families. Most mothers simply cannot be at the hospital as much as would probably be ideal for the infant. Two approaches are needed here. First, ways need to be found to help the mother be more available to her infant. This is particularly important when the mother is breast-feeding. Conceivably, as the therapeutic value of KC becomes more clear, government support will become available. Precedent appears in the broad-scale maternal leave systems provided in some countries (e.g., Sweden) and in the maternal stipends for child care and transportation provided in the grant funded by the U.S. Office of Education described by Gale et al. (1993). Community resources, such as government agencies, nongovernmental organizations, and volunteer groups, could become involved as well. Even given unlimited resources, however, the tolerance of individual mothers for being in the NICU must also be considered. Tolerance could be infinitely improved in an environment similar to the one described under facilitation.

The second approach involves considering who or what might substitute for the mother when she is not giving KC. The first step has already begun, in that fathers are becoming accepted as KC providers, with the mother receiving preferential access only if she is breast-feeding. This is a very recent development, at least in the United States. Now it is time to extend this opportunity to 1 or 2 other family members or close friends approved by the parents. This would be one way to respond to the suggestion by Kennell and Klaus that there "be a much stronger effort to bring grandparents and other supportive family members into the NICUs to help anxious, depleted, and bewildered parents through the long trying period of hospitalization" (1985, p. 275). During times when no KC provider is available or when the infant is unable to tolerate handling, the other developmentally oriented interventions described in this text, especially containment (Als et al., 1986, 1994; Buehler et al., 1995), are logical substitutes. This raises the interesting question of which of these interventions could be tolerated if KC could not, and vice versa.

PREDICTIONS AND RECOMMENDATIONS

Most KC trends in the United States have already been discussed, for example, the increasing number of documented benefits of KC, the heightened awareness of these benefits among health-care professionals and consumers of health care, and the spread of KC here and there across the nation. The prediction regarding these trends is that they will continue and intensify. In particular, the increasing number of documented benefits of KC leads to further predictions and recommendations.

The first prediction is that for most preterm infants, KC will become the standard of care throughout the world within 10 years. This is plausible because KC essentially sells itself through positive infant and parental responses and through monitoring of physiologic measures taken before, during, and after KC.

The second prediction is that it will become clear that the potential for cost reduction is enormous with KC, because of lower acuity in the hospital, earlier discharge home, and healthier long-term development. To date, cost reduction has been measured in only 1 published randomized clinical trial (RCT), the one by Sloan et al. (1994) in which the KC infants had less severe morbidity and costs were lower through 6 months of follow-up. Thus, RCTs with longer follow-up will be invaluable in addressing the cost-reduction issue. Another kind of KC cost reduction has been noticed as well. When mothers care for their infants in developing countries, a marked reduction is seen in the number of nurses needed to provide infant care (Bergman & Jürisoo, 1994; Davanzo, 1993; Levin, 1994).

Another prediction is that increased awareness of KC health benefits will lead parents to demand KC, if their requests for KC are refused. Thus, the ethics of withholding KC will become an issue for serious debate. The legal forms mentioned earlier may be sufficient to avoid problems in some cases, but where they are not, the conceivable ultimate outcome will be a malpractice suit brought by parents who were denied the opportunity to give KC.

Once health and cost-effectiveness are documented, the need to give as much KC as possible will become obvious, and government support, one hopes, will follow quickly for mothers who are willing. Basic support should include job protection, child care for older siblings, household care, and money to cover transportation, parking, meals, and "hoteling" at the hospital. If priorities must be established, first consideration should be given to mothers who breast-feed their infants. If for no other reason, there is a psychophysiological one: the higher the stress hormone cortisol in the mother's milk, the lower the IgA (Gröer, Humenick, & Hill, 1994), an important immune factor. Potentially then, the more the mother can be protected from stress, the more immunity protection she can provide to her infant through her breast milk. Another prediction is that families will be allowed to choose additional persons to help them give KC, and hospital staff will become comfortable about this practice, just as they are now becoming comfortable about fathers giving KC.

The first recommendation is to conduct well-designed and well-controlled RCTs as soon as possible to test the effectiveness of KC in developed countries. If effectiveness is found, then consensus conferences sponsored by WHO or the National Institutes of Health (NIH) (Wagner, 1994) and multisite RCTs should follow. A similar process is already underway in developing countries (Bureau of International Health, 1996). This respected process is the most reliable way to establish convincing scientific truth, which in turn is the optimal way to reach neonatologists and policy makers. Various subpopulations of infants need to be studied, including high acuity infants who are intubated, infants who are chronically ill with bronchopulmonary dysplasia, and 2 groups of infants drug-exposed *in utero*: those whose mothers are in rehabilitation programs and those whose mothers are not. In every RCT, interactions with gender, race, and feeding method should be evaluated.

The more mature preterm infants, who are reasonably healthy at birth and have the best chance for a normal outcome across the life span, should also be studied. In these trials, KC should begin at birth and be virtually continuous. Mothers and infants need to be watched vigilantly until the mothers know what to do, understand they must continue this kind of care for an indefinite number of days to maintain their infant in a healthy state, and can be counted on to accept this responsibility. Even infants who begin to grunt during the first 30 minutes can begin or continue KC, at least if they are between 32 and 36 weeks gestation, are healthy at birth, and are given warmed and humidified oxygen by hood until the grunting stops (Argote et al., 1991; Figure 6.3). The potential is great that these more mature preterm infants, if healthy at birth, do not need NICU care, provided they are given KC as just described. Bergman (personal communication, October 27, 1996) found this was also true for infants who are 31–33 weeks gestation (Bergman & Jürisoo, 1994). Thus, KC may be viewed as important not only *in* the NICU but for keeping some lower-risk preterm infants *out* of the NICU. However, RCTs are needed to test this hypothesis definitively, before widespread clinical use can begin (Silverman, 1985, 1992; Sinclair & Bracken, 1992).

All RCTs should continue KC after hospital discharge, because KC would be more powerful if continued into the home milieu. Two additional interventions would permit even earlier discharge and may increase and sustain the positive outcomes of KC: the Brooten nurse specialist transitional model, which provides continuity of caregiver between hospital and home (Brooten et al., 1986, 1995) and community-based interventions for ultimate follow-through and connectedness to the community. Further, RCTs must be used to assess the long-term effects of KC for two reasons: first, to estimate the full potential for health effectiveness, growth and development, and cost reduction; second, to learn whether the life span adverse effects of early maternal-infant separation, so well documented in animal models, may occur in humans as well.

CONCLUSIONS

The search continues for the ideal, comprehensive intervention to complement the medical and developmental advances reported for preterm infants over the past 30 years. KC has been widely used, and its safety even for small infants has been demonstrated. Nonetheless, more research on KC is needed to document effectiveness and cost reduction more definitively and to identify the mechanisms of its action. Further study is also needed to identify how KC can be, and whether it should be, used in conjunction with other developmental interventions and under what circumstances. These challenges increase in urgency as more sick infants survive and are cared for in even more technologically oriented units.

Acknowledgments

Preparation of this manuscript was supported by grants from the National Institute of Nursing Research, NIH (R01-NR02444 and 2R01 NR02444-04A1), and the Edward J. and Louise Mellen Foundation, Cleveland, OH.

The assistance of Linda Campbell and Meghan Moran in the preparation of this manuscript is gratefully acknowledged, as are the helpful comments of Nils Bergman, Maggie Cohea, Gay Gale, Susan Ludington, and Brigitte Syfrett on earlier versions of the manuscript.

Correspondence and requests for reprints should be sent to Gene Cranston Anderson, Ph.D., R.N., F.A.A.N., Mellen Professor of Nursing, Frances Payne Bolton School of Nursing, Case Western Reserve University, 10900 Euclid Avenue, Cleveland, OH 44106-4904. E-mail: gca@po.cwru.edu.

REFERENCES

Affonso, D., Bosque, E., Wahlberg V., & Brady, J. P. (1993a). Kangaroo care [Response to a letter to the editor]. *Neonatal Netw, 12(5),* 56–57.

Affonso, D., Bosque, E., Wahlberg V., & Brady, J. P. (1993b). Reconciliation and healing for mothers through skin-to-skin contact provided in an American tertiary level intensive care nursery. *Neonatal Netw, 12(3),* 25–32.

Affonso, D., Wahlberg, V., & Persson, B. (1989). Exploration of mothers' reactions to the kangaroo method of prematurity care. *Neonatal Netw, 7(6)*, 43–51.

Als, H., Lawhon, G., Brown, E., Gibes, R., Duffy, F. H., McAnulty, G., & Blickman, J. G. (1986). Individualized behavioral and environmental care for the very low birth weight preterm infant at high risk for bronchopulmonary dysplasia: neonatal intensive care unit and developmental care. *Pediatrics, 78(6)*, 1123–32.

Als, H., Lawhon, G., Duffy, F. H., McAnulty, G. B., Gibes-Grossman, R., & Blickman, J. G. (1994). Individualized developmental care for the very low-birth-weight preterm infant. *JAMA, 272*, 853–858.

Anderson, G. C. (1975). A preliminary report: severe respiratory distress in transitional newborn lambs with recovery following nonnutritive sucking. *J Nurse Midwifery, 20(2)*, 20–28.

Anderson, G. C. (1977). The mother and her newborn: mutual caregivers. *J Obstet Gynecol Neonatal Nurs (JOGNN), 6(5)*, 50–57.

Anderson, G. C. (1989a). Risk in mother-infant separation postbirth. *Image J Nurs Sch, 21*, 196–199.

Anderson, G. C. (1989b). Skin to skin: kangaroo care in Western Europe. *Am J Nurs 89*, 662–666.

Anderson, G. C. (1991). Current knowledge about skin-to-skin (kangaroo) care for preterm infants. *J Perinatol, 11*, 216–226.

Anderson, G. C. (1993). Kangaroo care [Letter to the editor]. *Neonatal Netw, 12(5)*, 56.

Anderson, G. C. (1995). Touch and the kangaroo care method. In T. Field (Ed.), *Touch in Early Development* (pp. 35–51). Mahwah, NJ: Erlbaum.

Anderson, G. C., Chang, H.-P., Behnke, M., Conlon, M., & Eyler, F. D. (1995). Self-regulatory mothering (SR) postbirth: effect on, and correlation between, infant crying and salivary cortisol. *Pediatr Res, 37(4)*, part 2 (Abstract 57, p. 12A).

Anderson, G. C., Marks, E. A., & Wahlberg, V. (1986). Kangaroo care for premature infants [published erratum appears in *Am J Nurs 86*, 1000]. *Am J Nurs, 86*, 807–809.

Anderson, G. C., Silvers, J. B., Miller, M., Singer, L., Yamashita, T., & Dowling, D. (1996–2000). Self-regulatory preterm infant care: adaptation postbirth. Grant number 2R01 NR02444-04A1. Bethesda, MD: National Institute of Nursing Research, National Institutes of Health.

Argote, L. A., Rey, H., Ludington, S., Medellín, G., Castro, E., & Anderson, G. (1991). Dificultad respiratoria transitoria y contacto piel a piel temprano como manejo. Memorias: 532. XVII Congreso Colombiano de Pediatria, Cali, Colombia, November (Abstract). English translation available from author.

Armstrong, H., & Kamau, M. (1986). Feeding low-birthweight babies. Co-produced by IBFAN and UNICEF (ESARO). [Videotape available from Tony Tirado, UNICEF, Division of Information, RTFSH9-F, 3 UN Plaza, New York, NY 10017.]

Baum, J. D., & Searls, D. (1971). Head shape and size of newborn infants. *Dev Med Child Neurol, 13*, 572–575.

Bergman, N. J., & Jürisoo, L. A. (1994). The "Kangaroo-method" for treating low birth weight babies in a developing country. *Trop Doct, 24*, 57–60.

Bosque, E. M., Brady, J. P., Affonso, D. D., & Wahlberg, V. (1995). Physiologic measures of kangaroo versus incubator care in a tertiary-level nursery. *J Obst Gynecol Neonatal Nurs, 24(3)*, 219–226.

Brigham & Women's Hospital. (1993). *Proceedings of the Eighth Annual Nursing Conference in Neonatology. Kangaroo Care: Changing Times and Emerging Trends.* Boston, MA: Author.

Brooten, D., Kumar, S., Brown, L. P., Butts, P., Finkler, S. A., Bakewell-Sachs, S., Gibbons, A., & Delivoria-Papadopoulos, M. (1986). A randomized clinical trial of early hospital discharge and home follow-up of very-low-birth-weight infants. *N Engl J Med, 315*, 934–939.

Brooten, D. A., Naylor, M., York, R., Brown, L., Roncoli, M., Hollingsworth, A., Cohen, S., Arnold, L., Finkler, S., Munro, B. H., & Jacobsen, B. S. (1995). Effects of nurse specialist transitional care on patient outcomes and cost: results of five randomized trials. *Am J Manag Care, 1*, 45–51.

Buehler, D. M., Als, H., Duffy, F. H., McAnulty, G. B., & Liederman, J. (1995). Effectiveness of individualized developmental care for low-risk preterm infants: behavioral and electrophysiologic evidence. *Pediatrics, 96*, 923–932.

Bureau of International Health. (1996). Workshop on Kangaroo Mother Care. Trieste, Italy, October 24–26.

Chan, J. S. L., Kelley, M. L., & Khan, J. (1993). The effects of a pressure relief mattress on postnatal head molding in very low birth weight infants. *Neonatal Netw, 12*, 19–22.

Charpak, N., Ruiz-Peláez, J. G., & Charpak, Y. (1994). Rey-Martinez kangaroo program: an alternative way of caring for low birth weight infants? One year mortality in a two cohort study. *Pediatrics, 94*, 804–810.

Christensson, K., Cabrera, T., Christensson, E., Uvnäs-Moberg, K., & Winberg, J. (1995). Separation distress call in the human infant in the absence of maternal body contact. *Acta Paediatr, 84*, 468–473.

Christensson, K., Siles C., Moreno, L., Belaustequi A., De La Fuente P, Lagercrantz H., Puyol P, & Winberg, J. (1992). Temperature, metabolic adaptation and crying in healthy full-term newborns cared for skin-to-skin or in a cot. *Acta Paediatr, 81*, 488–493.

Collins, S. (1993, March-April). Baby Stephanie: a case study in compassionate care. *Neonat Intens Care, 6*, 47–49.

Conlon M., & Anderson, G. C. (1990). Three methods of random assignment: comparison of balance achieved on potentially confounding variables. *Nurs Res, 39*, 376–379.

Curry, M. A. (1982). Maternal attachment behavior and the mother's self-concept: the effect of early skin-to-skin contact. *Nurs Res, 31(2)*, 73–78.

Davanzo, R. (1993). *Care of the low birth weight infants with the kangaroo method in developing countries. Guidelines for health workers.* Trieste, Italy: Bureau for International Cooperation in Maternal and Child Health, WHO Collaborating Centre for Maternal and Child Health, Istituto per l'Infanzia, Via dell' Istrud 65/1, 34137.

de Leeuw, R. (1986). The kangaroo method. *Vraagbak. Dev Workers, 14(4)*, 50–58.

de Leeuw, R., Colin, E. M., Dunnebier, E. A., & Mirmiran, M. (1991). Physiological effects of kangaroo care in very small preterm infants. *Biol Neonate, 59*, 149–155.

de Leeuw, R. (1992). History of the kangaroo care in the neonatal department of the Academic Medical Center, Amsterdam, Holland. In H. Martínez-Gómez & J. Aguilar (Eds.), *Primer Encuentro Internacional Programa Madre Canguro [First Internacional Conference on Mother Kangaroo Program]* (pp. 365–369). Bogotá, Colombia: UNICEF, Oficina Regional Para América Latina y el Caribe. [Available from UNICEF, 3 UN Plaza, New York, NY 10017.]

Drosten-Brooks, F. (1993). Kangaroo care: skin-to-skin contact in the NICU. *MCN Am J Matern Child Nurs, 18*, 250–253.

Färdig, J. A. (1980). A comparison of skin-to-skin contact and radiant warmers in promoting neonatal thermoregulation. *J Nurse Midwifery, 25(1)* 19–28.

Gale, G., Franck, L., Lund, C. (1993). Skin-to-skin kangaroo holding of the intubated premature infant. *Neonatal Netw, 12(6),* 49–57.

Gill, N. E., White, M. A., Anderson, G. C. (1984). Transitional newborn infants in a hospital nursery: from first oral cue to first sustained cry. *Nurs Res, 33(4),* 213–217.

Gloppestad, K. (1987). From separation to closeness: interviews with parents separated from their prematurely born infants [Videotape]. Oslo, Norway: National Hospital.

Gloppestad, K. (1995). Initial separation time between fathers and their preterm infants: comparison between two time periods. *Vard Nord Utvecki Forsk, 2, 15(2),* 10–17.

Graven, S. N. (1983). The University of Missouri Infant Development Unit and Program. *Zero to Three,* December, 12–13.

Gröer, M. W., Humenick, S., Hill, P. D. (1994). Characterization and psychoneuroimmunologic implications of secretory immunoglobulin A and cortisol in preterm and term breastmilk. *J Perinat Neonatal Nurs 7(4),* 42–51.

Hamelin, K., & Ramachandran, C. (1993). Kangaroo care. *Can Nurse,* 89(6), 15–17.

Harrison, L., & Klaus, M. H. (1994). Commentary: a lesson from eastern Europe. *Birth, 21(1),* 45–46.

IBFAN (International Baby Food Action Network). (1990). *Statement on Cups.* Copies available from IBFAN-Africa, PO Box 34308, Nairobi, Kenya.

Johanson, R. B., Spencer, S. A., Rolfe, P., Jones, P., & Malla, D. S. (1992). Effect of postdelivery care on neonatal body temperature. *Acta Paediatr, 81,* 859–863.

Kennell, J. H., & Klaus, M. H. (1985). Ethical considerations in the intensive care nursery. Commentary 2. In A. W. Gottfried, J. L. Gaiter, (Eds.), *Infant Stress Under Intensive Care. Environmental Neonatology* (pp. 271–277). Baltimore, MD: University Park Press.

Kriewall, T. J. (1982). Structural, mechanical, and material properties of fetal cranial bone. *Am J Obstet Gynecol, 143,* 07–714).

Kyenkya-Isabirye, M. (1992). UNICEF launches the Baby-Friendly Hospital Initiative. *MCN Am J Matern Child Nurs, 17,* 177–179.

Laine, A. M. (1987) Kangaroo care in Turku's University Hospital Pediatric Clinic. *Katilolehti, 92(5)* 171–176.

Lang, S., Lawrence, C. J., Orme, RL'E. (1994). Cup feeding: an alternative method of infant feeding. *Arch Dis Child, 71,* 365–369.

Lawrence, R. (1994). *Breastfeeding: A Guide for the Medical Profession.* St. Louis, MO: Mosby.

Legault, M., & Goulet, C. (1995). Comparison of kangaroo and traditional methods of removing preterm infants from incubators. *J Obst Gynecol Neonatal Nurs, 24(6),* 501–506.

Levin, A. (1994). The Mother-Infant Unit at Tallinn Children's Hospital, Estonia: a truly baby-friendly unit. *Birth, 21(1),* 39–44.

Levine, M. E. (1991). The conservation principles: a model for health. In K. M. Schaefer & J. B. Ponds (Eds.), *Levine's Conservation Model: A Framework for Nursing Practice* (pp. 1–11). Philadelphia: Davis.

Lind, J., Stern, L., & Wegelius, C. (1964/1974). Human fetal and neonatal circulation. In S. Z. Walsh, W. W. Meyer, & J. Lind, (Eds.), The Human Fetal and Neonatal Circulation (pp. 88–94). Springfield, IL: Thomas.

Ludington, S. M. (1995–1997). Pulmonary improvement in premature infants. Grant number 2R55 NR/OD02251–04. Bethesda, MD: National Institute of Nursing Research, National Institutes of Health.

Ludington, S. M. (1990). Energy conservation during skin-to-skin contact between premature infants and their mothers. *Heart Lung, 19(5),* 445–451.

Ludington-Hoe, S. M., Anderson, G. C., Simpson, S., Hollingsead, A., Rey, H., Argote, L. A., & Hosseini, B. (1993). Skin-to-skin contact beginning in the delivery room for Colombian mothers and their preterm infants. *J Hum Lact, 9,* 241–242.

Ludington-Hoe, S. M., Anderson, G. C., Swinth, J., Thompson, C., & Hadeed, A. J. (1994). Kangaroo care [Letter]. *Neonatal Netw, 13(4),* 61–62.

Ludington-Hoe, S. M., & Golant, S. K. (1993). *Kangaroo Care: The Best You Can Do to Help Your Preterm Infant.* New York: Bantam.

Ludington-Hoe, S. M., Hadeed, A. J., & Anderson, G. C. (1991). Physiologic responses to skin-to-skin contact in hospitalized premature infants. *J Perinatol, 11,* 19–24.

Ludington-Hoe, S. M., Hashemi, M. S., Argote, L. A., Medellin, G., & Rey, H. (1992). Selected physiologic measures and behavior during paternal skin contact with Colombian preterm infants. *J Dev Physiol, 18,* 223–232.

Ludington-Hoe, S. M., & Kasper, C. (1995). A physiologic method of monitoring premature infants. *J Nurs Meas, 3(1),* 13–29.

Ludington-Hoe, S. M., & Swinth, J. (1994). Abnormal breathing reduction in preterm infants during skin-to-skin contact (Abstract). *Infant Behav and Dev (Special ICIS Issue), 17,* 792.

Ludington-Hoe, S. M., Thompson C., Swinth, J., Hadeed, A. J., & Anderson, G. C. (1994). Kangaroo care: research results and practice implications and guidelines. *Neonatal Netw, 13(1),* 19–27.

Martínez-Gómez, H., & Aguilar, J. (Eds.). (1992). *Primer Encuentro Internacional Programa Madre Canguro [First International Conference on Mother Kangaroo Program].* Bogotá, Colombia, UNICEF, Oficina Regional Para Américana Latina y el Caribe. [Available for UNICEF, 3 UN Plaza, New York, NY 10017.]

Martínez-Gómez, H., Rey Sanabria, E., & Marquette, C. M. (1992). The mother kangaroo programme. *Int Child Health, 3,* 55–67.

McCloskey, J. M., & Bulechek, G. M. (1995). *Nursing Interventions Classification* (NIC) (2nd ed.). St. Louis, MO: Mosby.

McKenna, J., Thoman, E., Anders, T., Sadeh A., Schechtman, V., & Glotzbach, S. (1993). Infant-parent co-sleeping in an evolutionary perspective: implications for understanding infant sleep development and the sudden infant death syndrome. *Sleep, 16,* 263–282.

Meaney, M. J., Tannenbaum B., Francis, D., Bhatnagar, S., Shanks, N., Viau, V., O'Donnell, D., & Plotsky, P. (1994). Early environmental programming of hypothalamic-pituitary-adrenal responses to stress. *Sem Neurosci, 6,* 247–259.

Meier, P. (1988). Bottle-and-breast-feeding: effects on transcutaneous oxygen pressure and temperature in preterm infants. *Nurs Res, 37,* 36–41.

Meier, P. P., Engstrom, L. L., Mangurten, H. H., Estrada, E., Zimmerman, B., & Kopparthi, R. (1993). Breastfeeding support services in the Neonatal Intensive-Care Unit. *J Obst Gynecol Neonatal Nurs, 22,* 338–347.

Messmer, P. R., Wells-Gentry, J., Rodriguez, S., & Washburn, K. (1995). Mother's feelings on kangaroo care for their pre-term infants (pp. 243–250). In P. L. Munhall & V. M. Fitzsimmons (Eds.), *The Emergence of Women Into the 21st Century.* New York: NLN Press.

Moeller-Jensen, H., Hjort-Gregersen, K., Matthiessen, M., Vestergaard, H. F., & Jepsen, B. H. (1987). *The Kangaroo Method Used in Practice at the Hospital of Sønderborg, Denmark. Sygeplejersken.* English translation from Danish by Anne Larsen and Lotte Albret Wissing. Copenhagen: UNICEF.

Mondlane, R. P., de Graca, A. M. P., & Ebrahim, G. J. (1989). Skin-to-skin contact as a method of body warmth for infants of low birth weight. *J Trop Pediatr, 35,* 321–326.

Murdoch, D. R., & Darlow, B. A. (1984). Handling during neonatal intensive care. *Arch Dis Child, 59,* 957–961.

Nilsson, L. (1990). *A Child Is Born.* New York: Dell.

Odent, M. (1984). *Birth Reborn.* New York: Random House.

Ourth, L., Brown, K. B. (1961). Inadequate mothering and disturbance in the neonatal period. *Child Develop, 32,* 287–295.

Peabody, J. L., & Lewis, K. (1985). Consequences of newborn intensive care. In A. W. Gottfried & J. L. Gaiter (Eds.), *Infant Stress Under Intensive Care. Environmental Neonatology* (pp. 199–226). Baltimore, MD: University Park Press.

Pickler, R. H. (1993). Premature infant-nurse caregiver interaction. *Western J Nurs Res, 15,* 548–567.

Rapaport, L. (1965). The state of crisis: some theoretical considerations. In H. J. Parad (Ed.), *Crisis Intervention: Selected Readings.* (pp. 22–31). New York: Family Service Association of America.

Rey, E., & Martinez, H. (1983). *Manejo Racional del Niño Prematuro. Proceedings of the Conference I Curso de Medicina Fetal y Neonatal, Bogotá, 1981* (pp. 137–151). Bogotá, Colombia: Fundacion Vivar (Spanish). [Manuscript available in English from UNICEF, 3 UN Plaza, New York, NY 10017.]

Righard, L., & Alade, M. O. (1990). Effects of delivery room routines on success of first breast-feed. *Lancet, 336,* 1105–1107.

Righard, L., & Frantz, K. (1992). *Delivery Self-Attachment* [Videotape]. Sunland, CA: Geddes Productions.

Riordan, J. R., & Auerbach, K. G. (1993). Breastfeeding and human lactation. Boston: Jones & Bartlett.

Rosenberg, S., & Balmes, R. (1995). *Kangaroo Care: A Parent's Touch* [Videotape]. Chicago: Northwestern Memorial Hospital Media Services.

Schwirian, P. M., Eesley, T., & Cuellar, L. (1986). Use of water pillows in reducing head shape distortion in preterm infants. *Res Nurs Health, 9,* 203–207.

Silverman, W. A. (1985). *Human Experimentation. A Guided Step Into the Unknown.* New York: Oxford University Press.

Silverman, W. A. (1992). Foreword. In J. C. Sinclair & M. B. Bracken (Eds.), *Effective Care of the Newborn Infant.* New York: Oxford University Press. pp vii–viii.

Sims, C. I. (1988). Kangaroo care. *Mothering, 49,* 64–69.

Sinclair, J. C., & Bracken, M. B. (Eds.). (1992). *Effective Care of the Newborn Infant.* New York: Oxford University Press.

Sloan, N. L., Camacho, L. W. L., Rojas, E. P., & Stern, C. (1994). Kangaroo method: randomised controlled trial of an alternative method of care for stabilized low-birthweight infants. *Lancet, 344,* 82–785.

Sontheimer, D., Fischer, C. B., Scheffer, F., Kaempf, D., & Linderkamp, O. (1995). Pitfalls in respiratory monitoring of premature infants during kangaroo care. *Arch Dis Child, 72,* F115–F117.

Soukhanov, A. H. (1992). Word watch. *Atlantic, 270,* 4, 127.

Syfrett, E. B., Anderson, G. C., Behnke, M., Neu, J., & Hilliard, M. E. (1993a). Early and virtually continuous kangaroo care for lower-risk preterm infants: effect on temperature, breastfeeding, supplementation, and weight (Abstract). *Proceedings of the Biennial Conference of the Council of Nurse Researchers.* Washington, DC: American Nurses Association.

Syfrett, E. B., Anderson, G. C., Behnke, M., Neu, J., & Hilliard, M. E. (1993b). Kangaroo care for 34–36 week infants beginning in the delivery room: four infants and what we learned (Abstract). *Proceedings of the Eighth Annual Nursing Conference in Neonatology. Kangaroo Care: Changing Times and Emerging Trends.* Boston: Brigham & Women's Hospital.

U.S. Department of Health and Human Services, Division of Maternal and Child Health. (1985). *Follow-up Report: The Surgeon General's Workshop on Breastfeeding and Human Lactation.* Washington, DC: U.S. Government Printing Office, DHHS publication no. (HRS) D-MC 85-2.

Uvnäs-Moberg, K., Widström, A. M., Marchini, G., & Winberg, J. (1987). Release of GI hormones in mother and infant by sensory stimulation. *Acta Paediatr, 76,* 851–860.

Van Art, L. W, & Higgins, K. M. (1977). Three cases of an almost immediate therapeutic effect from sucking. *J Nurse Midwifery, 22(1),* 11.

Victor, L., & Persoon, J. (1994). Implementation of kangaroo care. A parent-health care team approach to practice change. *Crit Care Nurs Clin North Am, 6,* 891–895.

Wagner, M. (1994). *Pursuing the Birth Machine. The Search for Appropriate Birth Technology.* Kent, United Kingdom: ACE Graphics.

Wahlberg, V. (1991). The "Kangaroo method" and breastfeeding in low birth weight babies. *NU Nytt om U-landshälsovård, 5,* 23–27.

Wahlberg, V., Affonso, D., & Persson, B. (1992). A retrospective comparative study using the kangaroo method as a complement to standard incubator care. *Euro J Pub Health, 2(1),* 34–37.

Wallace, J., & Ridpath-Parker, J. (1993). Kangaroo care. *Qual Manag Health Care, 2(1),* 1–5.

Wegman, M. E. (1995). Annual summary of vital statistics—1994. *Pediatrics, 96,* 1029–1039.

Whitby, C., DeCates, C. R., & Roberton, N. R. C. (1982). Infants weighing 1.8–2.5kg: should they be cared for in neonatal units or postnatal wards? *Lancet, 1,* 322–325.

Whitelaw, A., (1986). Skin-to-skin contact in the care of very low birth weight babies. *Maternal Child Health, 7,* 242–246.

Whitelaw A., Heisterkamp, G., Sleath, K., Acolet, D., & Richards, M. (1988). Skin to skin contact for very low birthweight infants and their mothers. *Arch Dis Child, 63,* 1377–1381.

Whitelaw A., & Sleath, K. (1985). Myth of the marsupial mother: home care of very low birth weight babies in Bogotá, Colombia. *Lancet, 1,* 1206–1208.

WHO/PAH Interregional Conference on Appropriate Technology Following Birth, Trieste, Italy, 1985.

Widström, A.-M., Marchini, G., Matthiesen A.-S., Werner, S., Winberg, J., & Uvnäs-Moberg, K. (1988). Nonnutritive sucking in tube-fed preterm infants: effects on gastric motility and gastric contents of somatostatin. *J Pediatr Gastroenterol Nutr, 7,* 517–523.

Widström, A.-M., Ransjö-Arvidson, A. B., & Christensson, K. (1993). *Breastfeeding Is . . . Baby's Choice* [Videotape]. Stockholm: BGK Enterprises.

Widström, A.-M., Ransjö-Arvidson, A. B., Christensson, K., Matthiesen, A.-S., Winberg, J., & Uvnäs-Moberg, K. (1987). Gastric suction in healthy newborn infants: effects on circulation and developing feeding behavior. *Acta Paediatr Scand, 76,* 566–572.

Winberg, J., & Kjellmer, I. (1994). The neurobiology of infant-parent interaction in the newborn period. *Acta Pediatr,* Suppl, 397, 1–102.

Wolff, P. H. (1966). The causes, controls, and organization of behavior in the neonate. *Psychol Issues,* 5(17).

7

THE BREATHING BEAR AND THE REMARKABLE PREMATURE INFANT

EVELYN B. THOMAN

Several decades of research have provided very few answers and raised many more questions about how to provide nurturing care for the preterm infant. Interest has evolved from a focus on providing additional stimulation or reducing stimulation to an emphasis on involving the parents in providing social interaction for their infants.

The context for these changing interests has been a growing recognition of the complexity of the premature infant as well as the heterogeneity among these infants. We now realize that premature infants differ from the earliest age because of variations in medical and postnatal histories and that each has a unique development course, although with some commonalities with other preterm babies. As Forrest (1988) points out, "Individual neurodevelopmental outcome remains very difficult to accurately predict prospectively in the neonatal intensive care unit (NICU), and infants with apparently similar neonatal courses may develop remarkably differently. This repeated observation should be a source of caution and humility to those making critical neonatal care decisions" (p. 224). We would add, "and also to researchers whose goals are to provide evidence for the most effective forms of intervention."

Researchers now believe that interventions must be designed to be *developmentally appropriate*, the buzzword of interventionists of the 1990s. Assessing whether any specific intervention may be developmentally appropriate requires, first, an understanding of the neurodevelopmental course of infants born prematurely and, second, indices of deviation from this course by individual infants. Yet what constitutes optimal care is still debatable as shown by the wide variations in NICU practices across the country and the ambiguities and discrepancies in research findings in studies of various interventions.

This chapter addresses the neurodevelopmental course of premature infants so that developmentally appropriate interventions can be provided and describes a new intervention that meets the requirement of individualized environmental

161

enrichment. Self-regulation provides the guiding framework for this approach to understanding and caring for premature infants.

First, we examine the capabilities of preterm babies for endogenous (i.e., self-regulatory) controls as they are expressed in developing sleep/wake states. The behavioral states are a basic biological rhythm and an expression of neurobehavioral status. They provide the context for any intervention because they mediate stimulus input and modulate responsiveness to stimulation. In addition, the states constitute the outcome index for many studies of interventions.

In the second section of the chapter, we describe the Breathing Bear, an intervention that exemplifies the notion of self-regulation for premature infants. The bear is put in the crib (or isolette) for the infant to touch or cuddle with, and the bear's "breathing" acts as a source of gentle, rhythmic stimulation. The infant regulates the amount and temporal parameters of stimulation received by moving to or away from the bear—thus, stimulation is *optional*. Because the infant controls the stimulation and also because the bear's breathing rate is set to reflect one of the infant's own biological rhythms—quiet sleep (QS) respiration rate—the Breathing Bear is a developmentally appropriate form of environmental enrichment for premature infants throughout the preterm period.

We describe studies of premature infants with a Breathing Bear, indicating the responsiveness of infants when they can control input from their environment and the consequences of experience with the bear for their developing neuroregulatory controls.

From evidence presented for self-regulatory capabilities of premature infants, we propose a new perspective on the competence of premature infants and on intervention strategies for enriching their early environment. Preterm babies can participate in their environment and improve their developing neurobehavioral competence, facilitating their emerging role as social partners. Creating such opportunities is part of the challenge of devising developmentally appropriate caregiving for the vulnerable but remarkably able preterm infant.

SLEEP/WAKE STATES AS SELF-REGULATION

The sleep/wake states are a system of behaviors that express and serve a baby's endogenous needs. The states mediate the infant's perception of internal processes as well as external events, and they modulate the infant's responses to those events.

Overall, the state organization of premature infants is uneven. By full-term age, their state organization is apparently more mature than full-terms in some ways and less mature in others (Booth, Thoman, & Leonard, 1980; Holditch-Davis & Thoman, 1987). As examples, by term age, premature babies are alert more, are awake more, show more rapid eye movements in active sleep (AS), and have longer bouts of quiet sleep than full-term babies. These characteristics suggest that they are developmentally advanced, possibly because of their greater postnatal age. However, premature infants also show more sleep-wake transitions, and the quality of their quiet sleep is more fragmented by movements. These characteristics suggest immaturity or deviancy.

In addition, premature babies also cry less throughout the day than full-term infants over the early postterm weeks (Holditch-Davis & Thoman, 1987), despite numerous studies indicating that preterm infants are more irritable than full-term infants (Aylward, 1982; Friedman, Jacobs, & Werthmann, 1982; Michaelis et al., 1973). The two characterizations of premature infants are not contradictory, as their reported irritability is based on short-term observations of responsiveness to social or environmental stimuli, usually in the laboratory, whereas my and my colleagues' observations of infants indicate less total crying throughout the day in the home. The lesser crying overall and greater irritability in some circumstances is difficult to interpret with respect to developmental status. However, when and how much an infant cries has significant implications for development because crying plays a role in the parent-infant relationship (Acebo & Thoman, 1992; Hewson, Oberklaid, & Menahem, 1987; Hopkins & von Wulfften Palthe, 1987; Korner, 1974; Lester & Zeskind, 1982; Zeskind & Shingler, 1991).

Fullterm infants are capable of buffering themselves against stimulus overload by changing state. In stressful circumstances, they may enter the waking states of daze or drowse, or they can even go directly into quiet sleep, called *stress sleep* (Prechtl, 1965; Thoman & Whitney, 1990; Wolff, 1966). In preterm infants, even social stimulation can serve as a stressor and lead to physiological decompensation (Gorski, 1983). Thus, development of the capability of using stress sleep or other expressions of "active" use of state for stimulus regulation during the preterm period needs to be investigated.

A TAXONOMY OF BEHAVIORAL STATES IN INFANTS

The states in our classification system are assigned from observer judgments of an infant's behavior patterns, with special attention given to eyes, face, skin coloring, motility, muscle tone, vocalization, and breathing. Judgments are based on the quality and the overall patterning of behaviors. These distinctions can be reliably judged, and measures from such judgments reliably describe individual infants (Thoman, 1975a, 1975b, 1982, 1985; 1986; Thoman, Acebo, & Becker, 1983; Thoman, et al., 1979; Thoman & Becker, 1979; Thoman, Becker, & Freese, 1978; Thoman, Korner, & Kraemer, 1976).

The following 10 waking and sleeping states are termed the *primary states.* They can be reliably observed in premature infants as early as 29 weeks (Holditch-Davis, 1990) and in our studies in full-term infants at least throughout the first year of life (Acebo, 1987); Becker & Thoman, 1983; Booth et al., 1980; Holditch-Davis & Thoman, 1987; Pugsley, Acebo, & Thoman, 1988; Thoman, 1975a, 1975b, 1990; Thoman, Davis, & Denenberg, 1987; Thoman et al., 1976; Thoman & Pugsley, 1986; Thoman & Whitney, 1990). The state categories will be characterized very briefly by the most prominent clues, as they have been described in greater detail in previous published reports (Thoman, 1990; Thoman et al., 1987).

Awake States

Alert. Infant's eyes are open, bright, shining, and attentive. Baby may be quiescent or active.

Non-alert Waking. Infant may be motorically active and obviously awake. If the eyes are open, they are dull and unfocused.

Fuss. Low-level fuss sounds are made continuously or intermittently. Activity level may vary.

Cry. Intense vocalizations occur either singly or in succession, along with a high level of motor activity.

Transition States Between Sleep and Waking

Drowse. Eyes are either open and "heavy-lidded" or opening and closing slowly. Infant is relatively quiescent motorically.

Daze. Infant's eyes are open but glassy and immobile. Motor activity is usually low.

Sleep-Wake Transition. Infant shows behaviors of both wakefulness and sleep, with neither consistently predominating. This state usually occurs when the infant is spontaneously awakening from AS.

Sleep States

Active Sleep (AS). Infant's eyes are closed, and respiration is uneven and primarily costal in nature. Intermittent rapid eye movements (REMs), twitches of the extremities and gross body movements or body-jerks occur. Other state-related behaviors in AS include smiles, frowns, grimaces, mouthing, sucking, or mouth-puckering.

Quiet Sleep (QS) Eyes are closed. Respiration is relatively slow, regular, and abdominal in nature. A tonic level of motor tone is maintained. Motor activity is absent except for isolated single movements or startles or jerks. Another state-related behavior in QS is rhythmic mouthing, which may vary in intensity and may recur at about 1-minute intervals over a period of several minutes.

Transition State Within Sleep

Active-Quiet Transition Sleep. Infant is making the transition between the two sleep states and shows characteristics of both states, especially with respect to respiration, muscle tone, and small movements.

A Summary State Set

The following state-clusters encompass all 10 primary states and are often more appropriate for clinical and some research purposes. Each of these clusters has been demonstrated to show measurement reliability (Thoman, 1990).

Alert
Non-alert Waking
Fuss or Cry
Drowse, Daze, or Sleep-Wake Transition
Active Sleep
Quiet Sleep or Active-Quiet Transition Sleep

It is always important to note and record the state-related behaviors for AS and QS, as the motor behaviors indicate the baby's restlessness and the facial expressions indicate affect.

Procedures for Observing or Recording Infants' Sleep/Wake States

My colleagues and I have used two major procedures for our studies of infants' states. For one series of studies, 7-hour behavioral observations were made in the home, recording throughout the day the baby's state, using the categories already described. In addition to state, mother behaviors and other infant behaviors were recorded. During sleeping periods, respiration was recorded by means of a small pressure sensor under the crib pad, connected to an analog recorder, which was turned on whenever the infant was in the crib (Thoman et al., 1979).

For another series of studies, we have used a procedure developed in this laboratory for sleep/wake monitoring, the Home Monitoring System (HMS), which is totally non-intrusive. A pressure-sensitive mattress pad is placed in the infant's crib, and 24 hours of motility from respiration and body movements is recorded on the single channel of a small recorder. Thus, it is possible to monitor the baby continuously without instrumentation (Thoman & Glazier, 1987; Thoman et al., 1986b; Thoman & Pugsley, 1986). In the laboratory, the recordings are computer-scored for AS, QS, active-quiet transition sleep, sleep-wake transition, and waking.

Both procedures permit naturalistic study of the states of infants. Behavioral observations permit recording of the full range of sleep and waking states as well as state-related behaviors, which include types of movements, REMs, vocalizations, and facial expressions. The automated recordings make it possible to collect continuous 24-hour data. Thus, the two kinds of recordings provide overlapping but differing information on infants' regulatory controls for state.

Early State Characteristics Are Related to Later Developmental Status

A taxonomy is relevant only if it is useful. Findings from both full-term and prematurely born infants, recorded in the home, will be summarized to indicate state measures that have proved to be indices of subtle central nervous system (CNS) dysfunction at an early age with serious implications for later developmental status.

A State Stability Index

Using behavioral observations, we found that inconsistent state patterning over successive weekly observations over postnatal weeks 2 to 5 in full-term infants indicated later developmental dysfunction (Thoman et al., 1981). A State Stability Index was derived to describe the degree of state consistency over observations for an individual infant. Briefly, the distribution of an infant's sleep and waking states within an observation is determined as the basis for a state profile obtained for each weekly observation. Then a quantitative measure of consis-

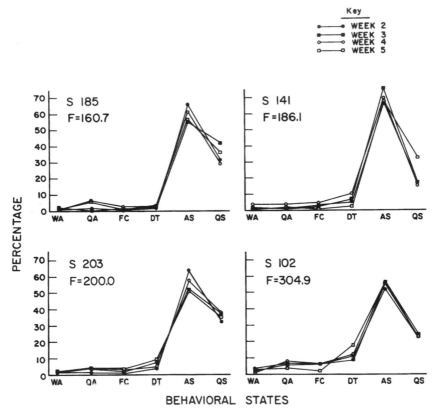

Figure 7.1. Weekly behavioral state profiles for four infants with high State Stability scores. Along with the X-axis are the behavioral states, the Y-axis is the percentage of time spent in each state. WA, waking active; QA, quiet alert; FC, fuss or cry; DT, drowse or transition: AS, active sleep; QS, quiet sleep. (●) Week 2, (■), Week 3, (○) Week 4, (□) Week 5.

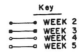

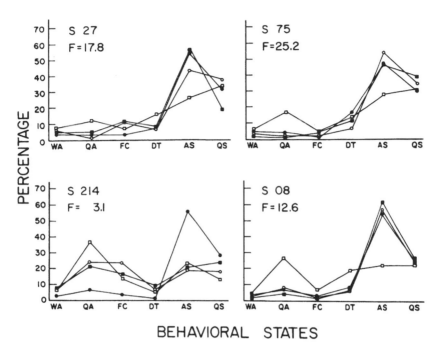

Figure 7.2. Weekly behavioral state profiles for four infants with low State Stability scores. Along with the X-axis are the behavioral states, the Y-axis is the percentage of time spent in each state. WA, waking active; QA, quiet alert; FC, fuss or cry; DT, drowse or transition: AS, active sleep; QS, quiet sleep. (●) Week 2, (■), Week 3, (○) Week 4, (□ Week 5.

tency of these profiles over weeks can be calculated using an analysis of variance (ANOVA), yielding a single state stability score (F = mean square for states/ mean square for states × weeks) for each infant for the successive observations. This measure of *consistency in state profiles* over successive observations depicts a form of temporal organization in states quite different from temporal sequence, recurrence time, or cyclicity. I will describe these more traditional indices of temporal structure later.

To illustrate the State Stability Index, Figure 7.1 presents the 4-week state profiles for 4 infants who were very stable over the weekly observations (despite variations of schedules of activities in the home), and Figure 7.2 presents the 4-week profiles for 4 very unstable infants (one was later found to be severely retarded and one died of Sudden Infant Death Syndrome) [SIDS]. The relatively disparate patterning of states over weeks is apparent in these 2 groups of infants. However, as seen in Figure 7.2, there is evidence for a remarkable degree of organization over time in even the most inconsistent subjects.

In a study of 22 full-term infants during the early postterm weeks, the 4 infants with the lowest State Stability Scores had the following outcomes: 1 infant developed aplastic anemia at 30 months of age; 1 showed infantile seizure at 6 months and became severely retarded; 1 died of SIDS at 3.5 months; and one became seriously hyperactive (Thoman et al., 1981). Of those infants with low mental scores, none had state stability scores above the median for the group. All of the infants were considered normal at the time of the early observations. Thus, instability in the state system of individual infants during the early weeks has major implications for later developmental status.

Premature babies at a comparable early age are capable of consistency in state patterning that does not differ significantly from that of full-term infants. Tynan (1986), using the State Stability Index for preterm infants, found that those who later showed serious dysfunction had the lowest scores on this measure. Accordingly, it is reasonable to conclude that the capabilities and incapacities of premature infants are revealed by this measure of state organization.

Characteristics of Siblings of SIDS Infants

As indicated in the previous section, 1 subject in our longitudinal study died of SIDS at 3 months. The extensive data on this baby's sleep/wake states and respiration indicated a number of deviations from the group (Thoman, et al., 1988). First, as already described, the baby had an extremely low state stability score. In addition, the baby had markedly deviant respiratory characteristics, including relatively fast and irregular respiration rates. Most dramatic was the finding of apnea frequencies markedly *lower* than any other baby's in the group, as well as an absence of any prolonged apneas (Thoman, Miano, & Freese, 1978). This result was contrary to the prevailing emphasis on apneas as placing infants at risk for SIDS. However, a "deficit" of apneas, as well as an excess, is now recognized by researchers as constituting a deviant respiratory pattern.

Three siblings of SIDS (SSIDS) infants were studied in the home using the 7-hour observations. Two of the infants showed normal sleep and respiratory characteristics, and they were predicted to develop without respiratory dysfunction. In contrast, the 3rd infant showed a pattern of deviancies similar to the SIDS infant; and at 4 months, she had prolonged apneic episodes, requiring resuscitation on 2 occasions. These results are consistent with the notion of subtle CNS dysfunction from the time of birth in infants who are vulnerable to SIDS (Valdes-Depena, 1982).

Prediction of Developmental Outcome From the First Postnatal Day

Using the automated HMS, described in a previous section on recording procedures, we recorded the sleep of newborn infants throughout their postnatal stay in the hospital. A number of sleep measures were found to be related to later developmental status: lower mental scores were predicted from day 1 recordings by longer mean sleep periods, longer longest-sleep-periods, less sleep-wake transition, and more arousals during QS (Ar/QS). Fewer relationships were found on postnatal day 2 (Freudigman & Thoman, 1993).

With the exception of the Ar/QS variable, the direction of the relationships on day 1 were contrary to the developmental course for these variables. We interpreted the results to indicate that sleep characteristics on the first postnatal day reflect a response to the stress of the birth process and that those infants who show the greatest deviation are most vulnerable. These results suggested that infants' sleep characteristics during the first postnatal day provide uniquely sensitive indices of later neurobehavioral functioning.

Prediction of Developmental Disabilities in Premature Infants

Using the HMS, we recorded the sleep/wake states of 100 premature infants in the home for 24-hour periods when they were 1, 2, 3, 4, and 5 weeks postterm (Whitney & Thoman, 1993). At 3 years of age, the babies were classified into one of four groups: (1) those who were normal, (2) those with neurodevelopmental disabilities, (3) those with physical problems, and (4) those with minor mental delay.

Profiles of state measures were formed from the following state variables: the amount of waking, AS, and QS, the mean AS bout length, the mean QS bout length, QS slope (developmental rate over the 5 weeks), AS slope, the longest sleep period, and the State Stability Index. The profiles for each of the groups with abnormal developmental outcome differed significantly from each other and from the group of normal infants. The profile measures predicted better for individuals than did clinical risk factors. These findings indicate that specific forms of later disabilities in premature infants are expressed in differential organization of sleep states during the earliest postterm period when developmental dysfunction is not yet apparent.

A Systems View of States and Their Adaptive Role

A baby's state system functions in relation to both brain and the environment at different levels of an hierarchical organization (Thoman, 1986). At each level, states play a role in assuring stability, plasticity, and continuity. Accordingly, we have proposed (Thoman et al., 1983) that state organization, as well as the infant's interactions with caregivers, can be viewed within general systems theory (GST), which is concerned with problems of organized complexity (Bertalanffy, 1933, 1968); Weiss, 1969, 1971). Bertalanffy (1933) proposed that any theory of development must be a systems theory, applicable to social relationships as well as other levels of biological organization. The characteristics of system dynamics are these: (1) there is ongoing feedback within the system, (2) the system functions to maintain its own equilibrium, and (3) there are simultaneous interactions of complex variables (Thoman, 1990). Clearly these criteria fit the states as a behavioral system.

These notions are relevant to consideration of any intervention for preterm infants. More specifically, they apply to the use of sleep/wake states as indices of effectiveness of the Breathing Bear intervention.

THE BREATHING BEAR INTERVENTION AND THE PREMATURE INFANT'S CAPABILITY FOR SELF-REGULATING STIMULATION: EFFECTS ON ORGANIZATION OF STATES, LEARNING, AND AFFECT

A major concern for the development of premature infants is each child's biological and behavioral capabilities for social interchange. However, caregivers face a dilemma because it is not always possible to provide parenting for preterm infants, especially while they need to be in an isolette. Furthermore, parenting is not always appropriate. Gorski (1983) reported subtle as well as gross behavioral and physiologic distress following close social interaction in preterm infants. This reaction occurs in part because these babies are less able than more mature infants to signal when stimulation is becoming overwhelming (DiVitto & Goldberg, 1979). In addition, they have fewer neurological regulatory controls that would enable them to inhibit costly responses to excessive demands or poorly timed stimuli from the environment (DiVitto, & Goldberg, 1979; Gorski et al., 1983).

The "breathing" teddy bear was designed as a surrogate mother or companion for prematures, which addresses this dilemma. The bear is 15 inches high, approximately the size of a 35-week preterm infant, and it is made to "breathe" by means of a pump located outside the crib that is connected to a bladder in the bear's torso via a plastic hose. The pump is very quiet and it makes the bear breathe with a smooth sinusoidal motion like that of a healthy full-term baby. The motion of the bear's body is a source of gentle, rhythmic stimulation for the infant.

The breathing bear eliminates over-stimulation because contact with it is controlled by the infant—the bear is placed in the isolette so the infant can touch and cuddle with it or move away. Thus, the infant regulates the amount and duration of stimulation. In addition, the stimulation provided by the bear is individualized for the infant it is with because the bear's "breathing" rate is based on the infant's own respiration rate during QS.

In the sections that follow, we discuss the issues for premature care addressed with this intervention. Then we summarize our studies of the Breathing Bear to indicate the capability of premature infants for self-regulating stimulation and to describe the consequences of experience with the bear for the developing neuroregulatory controls of these vulnerable infants.

Conceptual Bases for the Bear

Several theoretical considerations led to the design of a surrogate companion for premature infants (Thoman, 1993). The notion that premature infants should be able to choose to make contact with a source of rhythmic stimulus derived from findings demonstrating that newborn rat pups will seek contact with a warm, pulsating mother surrogate (Thoman & Arnold, 1968). Given that the newborn rat is similar to the human premature in amount of brain growth at birth compared to that in adulthood (Himwich, 1972) and that these altricial animals can make such a biologically relevant choice, we could reasonably expect such competence in the prematurely born human infant.

The hypotheses for the bear as a potential source of stimulation for prematures were these: (1) that the babies would prefer a breathing bear to a non-breathing one, (2) that premature infants would be capable of expressing this preference by mobilizing their motor activity to achieve contact with the bear, and (3) that such an experience with optional rhythmic stimulation should facilitate neurodevelopmental processes. The latter expectation also derived from the animal research: a stimulating mother surrogate was found to be necessary for the growth and survival of animals separated from their mother.

Evidence That Premature Infants Can Organize Their Motor Movements for an Approach Response

Our first study was designed to test these expectations (Thoman & Graham, 1986). Groups of premature infants 32 to 34 weeks conceptional age (CA) were given the opportunity to self-regulate contact with a Breathing Bear (BrBr) or a non-Breathing Bear (N-BrBr), while a third group of infants had no bear (N-Br) in the isolette. The Breathing Bear's breathing rate was reset every 3 days after observing the infant's breathing during a period of QS.

All infants were continuously monitored using time-lapse video recording with a camera placed directly over the isolette. From the videotapes, it was possible to score whether the baby was in contact with the bear and the occurrence of QS. To score contact in the N-Br condition, the space occupied by a bear in the isolette was covered on the video screen by a paper cutout (called a *shadow bear*), thus permitting us to obtain a baseline measure of the amount of chance contact babies had with that area of the crib.

We found that with only 2 weeks of exposure to this form of optional stimulation, infants spent far more time in contact with the Breathing Bear than did infants in either of the other two groups (Thoman & Graham, 1986). Subsequent studies have replicated this finding (Thoman & Ingersoll, 1989; Thoman, Ingersoll, & Acebo, 1991; Thoman, & Ingersoll, 1993; Ingersoll & Thoman, 1994; Thoman et al., 1995). The data confirmed our expectations that the Breathing Bear is an attractive, preferred stimulus for premature infants and that they have the competence to seek and achieve contact with it and thus to regulate the duration of their stimulation.

Viewing the videotapes at the time-lapse speed clearly indicated the infants' ability to move themselves about to establish physical contact with the bear—with their legs, limbs, head, or body. The possibility of overstimulation, with its attendant risks, is minimized by making the Breathing Bear continuously available but not imposed on the infant. At the same time, the bear enables the infants to "exercise" and develop their self-regulating capabilities.

Evidence for Entrainment

Another theoretical issue given serious consideration was the rhythm at which the bear would breathe. With no clear guide in the literature as to choice of rate, we felt that one of the baby's own biological rhythms would be most appropriate, based on the principles of entrainment (Abraham & Shaw, 1982;

Gander et al., 1984; Kronauer et al., 1982; Winfree, 1967). Abraham and Shaw point out that the closer the entraining frequency is to the fundamental frequency of the subject, the more optimal the conditions for the entrainment process. They also posit that "the phases need not be entrained, only the frequencies" (1982, p. 175). Thus, it is not necessary for the baby to breathe synchronously with the bear for the bear's regular "breathing" to entrain the baby's more irregular sleep and breathing patterns.

Evidence to support this expectation was obtained from 2-hour respiration recordings (Ingersoll and Thoman, 1994) made by means of a sensor pad placed under the infants, connected to a small paper-chart recorder. The analog motility signals can be reliably scored for the sleep states, and the regularity of respiration during QS can be judged on a 4-point scale (Thoman & Tynan, 1979; Thoman & Zeidner, 1979). This scoring can be accomplished with high interjudge reliability and with significant measurement reliability. Premature infants who had the bear for a 2-week period showed greater regularity of respiration during QS (Thoman and Ingersoll, 1993). This finding supports the notion that the Breathing Bear entrains the infants' respiration patterns.

Evidence from other studies, although more indirect, also supports the notion of entrainment from the bear. The sleep/wake states during the first postterm weeks were recorded using the automated HMS, which permits nonintrusive recording for 24-hour periods in the infant's crib (Thoman & Whitney, 1989). The procedure was the same as that described earlier in the section on sleep recording procedures. We found that the BrBr babies showed a greater amount of QS over this age range than N-BrBr babies (Thoman & Pugsley, 1986).

Evidence for Learning

Entrainment is one form of learning. We also investigated the possibility that the Breathing Bear would serve as a positive reinforcer for instrumental learning. For this purpose, the change in the latency to achieve contact following a caregiving intervention was correlated with the change in the amount of contact with the bear over the 2-week intervention period from 33 to 35 weeks CA. These measures were significantly correlated for the BrBr babies ($r = -.64$, $df = 19$, $p < .01$), but not for the babies with the N-BrBr babies ($r = -.07$, $df = 20$, ns). Thus, only for the BrBr babies, the increased amount of contact over the 2 weeks was associated with a decreased latency to make contact with the bear.

It is important to note that the changes in latency and contact for the Breathing Bear infants were not attributable to greater wakefulness at the later age, as both groups of infants showed a similar decrease in wakefulness over the 2 weeks. Although the BrBr babies showed more prolonged bouts of contact, their shorter latencies were not correlated with more prolonged bouts of contact with the bear. Thus, the increased contact with the bear over weeks did not reflect simply prolonged maintenance of contact following instances when the infants may have touched the bear by chance.

By demonstrating the premature's capability for "seek-find-touch" behaviors, studies of the Breathing Bear intervention have provided the first demonstration

of instrumental learning in preterm infants. At the same time, they have provided evidence for the basic capability of preterm infants for organized motor
behaviors that have received little attention.

Evidence for Facilitation of Neurobehavioral Development

One could argue that the increased QS (already described) both during the
preterm period and the postterm weeks indicates more advanced state organization in the BrBr babies. Additional findings indicate facilitation of neurobehavioral development by the experience with the bear.

The BrBr babies show not only greater regularity of QS respiration (already
described) but also slower respiration rates in both AS and QS: in AS, the mean
rate was 59.4 in the BrBr babies and 60.0 in the N-BrBr babies; in QS, 53.3
in the BrBr babies and 56.3 in the N-BrBr babies. Over both states, the difference is significant ($F = 11.806$, $df = 1,28$, $p <.01$). Since respiration rates
decline over age during the early months, this difference suggests that the development of neural controls for respiration has been facilitated by the experience with the bear.

Arousal movements in QS were lower in the preterm BrBr babies than the
N-BrBr babies. This variable indicates the degree to which QS is fragmented,
probably due to a lack of CNS inhibitory controls. Arousals in QS in newborn
full-term babies have been related to later mental delay (Freudigman & Thoman,
1993). Premature babies generally show greater fragmentation than full-term
infants during the early postterm weeks (Booth et al., 1980). Taken together,
these findings indicate that the decreased frequency of arousals in QS is another
indication of neurobehavioral facilitation by the bear intervention.

Evidence for Positive Affect Associated with the Breathing Bear

Approach responses to the bear provided clear evidence that the bear has a
positive valence for the infants. In our most recent study (Thoman et al., 1995),
we found evidence for more positive affect in the BrBr babies.

For that study, the sleep/wake states and state-related behaviors were observed for a 2-hour period after the infants graduated to an open crib. The BrBr
babies showed more smiles and fewer grimaces during sleep and less crying
during wakefulness than the N-BrBr babies. Thus, the difference in affect is
expressed both in sleep and wakefulness. Not only positive reinforcement from
the bear but also the opportunity for the babies to control an aspect of their
environment may account for more smiles and less crying.

Considerable evidence suggests that an intervention that increases positive
affect in infants is important for their neurobehavioral development. Papousek
and collaborators (Janos & Papousek, 1977; Papousek, Papousek, & Harris,
1984) have emphasized the central role of emotion in learning processes. Like-
wise, Prensky (1978) argues that stress is not optimal for brain growth.

We propose that more attention to positive affective expressions in premature infants may provide clues to events that may support or facilitate their development.

IMPLICATIONS OF THE SELF-REGULATION CAPABILITIES OF PREMATURES FOR THEIR EARLY CAREGIVING

The facet of self-organization that has received least attention is the premature infant's positive affect. An opinion still prevails among researchers (an opinion not heard from NICU nurses) that immature babies, even at full term, are devoid of feelings or expressions of emotion but are able only to cry or be quiescent. We have argued that newborns, even those born prematurely, experience a range of human feelings (Thoman & Acebo, 1984). Because language and mature motor capabilities are not available in early infancy, affects at this stage of life cannot be defined using operational definitions appropriate for study of emotions at older ages. However, neurophysiological, physical, and behavioral studies at the human and animal levels (Smotherman & Robinson, 1987) strongly support the view that the more complex emotions of later ages have their antecedents in affects of the fetus or premature infant as well as the full-term newborn infant. Furthermore, "most mammals are biologically pretuned to produce and to respond to expressive movement patterns and gesticulations which conform to basic biological rhythms" (Newson, 1974, p. 253), as these are expressed in emotion.

Such a view of early affect has implications for the importance of learning opportunities that interventions can provide for premature infants. The BrBr experience is a special case of learning with a positive reinforcer. Virtually any NICU nurse will confirm that the premature babies in their care come to anticipate and respond to impending interventions that are regularly necessary— and typically stressful or distressful. A major contribution of the Breathing Bear intervention is that the babies can learn about a feature of the environment that is consistently available and that elicits *positive affect*.

Implications for later development as a consequence of such an early experience can be only speculative at this time. Much has been written about older babies with respect to the importance of having early opportunities to develop contingency connections between the baby's own behavior and environmental events (Mahrer, Levinson, & Fine, 1976; Moss & Robson, 1968). As an example, the emergence of "wanting to do it oneself" has been proposed as a precursor of achievement motivation (Geppert & Kuster, 1983). The notion is one of infant-centeredness (White, 1972), which is in contrast to the predominant tendency of caregiving figures to assume completely the role of initiator and controller. We propose that it is important for even premature infants to have opportunities for control over their environment (Crandall, 1965; Moore, 1967) and to see the consequences of their own behavior (Crandall, 1965; Groos, 1908). Such experience can permit them to acquire some sense of environmental mastery (Ainsworth, 1967; Lewis & Goldberg, 1965; Mahrer et al., 1976).

Also, research with older babies has suggested that early positive learning experiences can influence a baby's later tolerance for aversive experiences. Purportedly, these experiences can serve to "inoculate" the baby against stress (Carlson & Masters, 1986). The Breathing Bear offers an opportunity to explore these principles in terms of effects on later behavior.

CONCLUDING COMMENTS

Despite the stresses of early and precipitous departure from the uterine environment and medical interventions necessary to assure survival, premature infants are remarkably well-organized individuals. New findings continue to reveal more about the nature of their organization. The research progress in this area suggests a parallel with the history of discoveries of capabilities of full-term babies during earlier decades. Once, newborn babies were claimed incapable of learning because of central neural limitations. From the time that Mavis Gunther (1961) made her dramatic demonstration of learning in the neonate, an enormous body of research has accumulated, which indicates that, from the time of birth, a full-term baby is prepared for action, interaction, and modification of behavior. We now recognize that these neurobehavioral capabilities for self-organization and interaction serve to assure a baby's adaptation to the environment and effective functioning as a social partner.

The research reported here and that of many other researchers is beginning to provide information on the developing neurobehavioral characteristics of premature infants. Clearly, the premature infant is a person with individual needs, capabilities, and responsiveness, and these change rapidly with age, especially during the preterm period. Much more research will be required before we are to fully understand the developmental processes of these infants and how they vary with gestational age at birth, during the medical course, and at postnatal age. Such information will be the basis for assessing the impact of any caregiving regimen on these processes. These issues are compounded by the survival of ever smaller infants because of advances in medical technology. Meanwhile, premature babies must be cared for, in the most humane and sensitive ways possible.

From this perspective, the available evidence for self-regulatory capabilities highlights the importance of "tuning in" to a premature infant before, during, and after any necessary medical or caregiving procedure. Our data suggest that the states of sleep and wakefulness provide the most prominent behavioral "cues" for tuning in to the baby, or even when to tune in—for example, an infant in QS is presenting a behavioral "do not disturb" sign, which merits respect whenever possible, whereas a smile in AS says, "I am pleased by whatever is going on." Indications of affect are expressed more frequently during AS than in wakefulness. This is significant because infants spend much more time in AS. The importance of positive affect and providing positive experiences for premature infants cannot be overemphasized (Thoman, 1981a, 1981b, 1985; Thoman & Acebo, 1984).

In view of the profound facilitative effects of the simple intervention provided by the Breathing Bear, we propose that most, if not all, premature infants would benefit by having their own Breathing Bear. Since stimulation from the bear is contingent on the infants' movements, this proposition applies to preterm infants after they have become physiologically stable and their movements are not restricted for purposes of medical care.

The next question, accordingly, is whether the same principles that assure the bear's benefits for stable premature babies may also be applicable at an earlier period, when such infants are even more fragile, or for those who have persisting serious health problems. Our objective is to investigate whether very gentle contact and rhythmic, individualized stimulation may also benefit the sick preterm infant, especially during the earliest postnatal period when such babies have to be immobilized for medical reasons. This direction for research is guided by the circumstance that ever smaller prematurely born infants are surviving because so much can be done for them medically, while so little can be done to facilitate their thriving. The bear, with modifications in design (such as smaller size!) and procedure for use may serve this function. The plan is to place the bear in contact with the babies for brief periods of time, particularly following stressful caregiving interventions. Physiological and behavioral assessment of the infants' responses to the intervention can, and should, be monitored to determine the efficacy of this form of additional stimulation for the most vulnerable infants. Then, when these premature babies become physiologically stable, the bear offers a unique opportunity for them to participate in their own therapeutic intervention, even while their experiences continue to be dominated by stressful reinforcers, as a medical necessity.

In conclusion, it is important to note a special advantage of the bear, namely that, as an intervention, it makes no additional demands on nursing staff. Some interventions have been introduced into the NICU, only to disappear because of time pressures in the nursery or because they are stressful for some infants.

While the breathing bear requires no time and attention from the caregivers, it provides a baby with constancy (always there), consistency (a regular rhythm), reassurance (the baby's own biological rhythm), positive reinforcement (soothing stimulation), and companionship (body contact). It is no wonder that babies who have had a breathing bear are happier—as suggested by their more positive affective behaviors. It is reasonable to speculate that such an experience should prepare them to be more positive and adaptive as social partners when they go home.

REFERENCES

Abraham, R. H., & Shaw, C. D. (1982). *Dynamics—The Geometry of Behavior. Part 1: Periodic Behavior.* In R. H. Abraham (Ed.), *The Visual Mathematics Library.* Santa Cruz: Aerial Press.

Acebo, C. (1987). *Naturalistic Observations of Mothers and Infants: Description of Mother and Infant Responsiveness and Sleep-Wake State Development.* Ph.D. diss., University of Connecticut.

Acebo, C., & Thoman, E. B. (1992). Crying as a social behavior. *Infant Mental Health Journal, 13 (1)*, 67–82.

Ainsworth, M. D. S. (1967). *Infancy in Uganda: Infant Care and the Growth of Love*. Baltimore: Johns Hopkins University Press.

Aylward, G. P. (1982). Forty-week full-term and preterm neurologic differences. In L. P. Lipsitt & T. M. Field (Eds.), *Infant Behavior and Development: Perinatal Risk and Newborn Behavior* (pp. 67–83). Norwood, NJ: Ablex.

Becker, P. T., & Thoman, E. B. (1983). Organization of sleeping and waking states in infants: consistency across contexts. *Physiology and Behavior, 31*, 405–410.

Bertalanffy, L. von (1933). *Modern Theories of Development: An Introduction to Theoretical Biology*. London: Oxford University Press.

Bertalanffy, L. von (1968). *General Systems Theory*. New York: Brazilier.

Booth, C. L., Thoman, E. B., & Leonard, H. L. (1980). Sleep states and behavior patterns in preterm and fullterm infants. *Neuropediatrics, 11*, 354–364.

Carlson, C. R., & Masters, J. C. (1986). Inoculation by emotion: effects of positive emotional states on children's reactions to social comparison. *Developmental Psychobiology, 22*, 760–765.

Crandall, V. C. (1965). Differences in Parental Antecedents of Internal-External Control in Children and in Young Adulthood. Paper presented at meeting of Society for Research in Child Development, Minneapolis.

DiVitto, B., & Goldberg, S. (1979). The effects of newborn medical status on early parent-infant interaction. In T. M. Field, A. M. Sostek, S. Goldberg, & H. H. Shuman (Eds.), *Infants Born at Risk: Behavior and Development* (pp. 311–332). New York: SP Medical and Scientific Books.

Forrest, C. B. (1988). Neuro-Developmental Outcome in Low Birth Weight Infants: The Role of Developmental Intervention. In R. Guthrie (Ed.), *Neonatal Intensive Care Clinics in Critical Care Medicine, Vol. 13*. Churchill Livingston.

Freudigman, K. A., & Thoman, E. B. (1993). Newborn sleep during the first postnatal day: an opportunity for assessment of vulnerability. *Pediatrics, 92*, 373–379.

Friedman, S. L., Jacobs, B. S., & Wethmann, M. W. (1982). Preterms of low medical risk: spontaneous behaviors and soothability at expected date of birth. *Infant Behavior and Development, 14*, 490–498.

Gander, P. H., Kronauer, R. E., Czeisler, C. A., & Moore-Ede, M. C. (1984). Modeling the action of zeitgebers on the human circadian system: comparisons of simulations and data. *American Physiological Society, 247*, R418–R426.

Geppert, U., & Kuster, U. (1983). The emergence of "wanting to do it oneself: a precursor of achievement motivation." *International Journal of Behavioral Development, 6*, 355–369.

Gorski, P. A. (1983). Premature infant behavioral and physical responses to caregiving interventions in the intensive care nursery. In J. Call, E. Galenson, & R. Tyson (Eds.), *Frontiers of Infant Psychiatry* (pp. 256–263). New York: Basic Books.

Gorski, P. A., Hole, W. T., Leonard, C. H., & Martin, J. A. (1983). Direct computer recording of premature infants and nursery care: distress following two interventions. *Pediatrics, 72(2)*, 198–202.

Groos, K. (1908). *The Play of Men*. New York: Appleton-Century-Crofts.

Gunther, M. (1961). Infant behavior at the breast. In B. M. Foss (Ed.), *Determinants of Infant Behaviour*. London: Methuen.

Hewson, P., Oberklaid, F., & Menahem, S. (1987). Infant colic, distress, and crying. *Clinical Pediatrics, 2*, 69–75.

Himwich, W. A. (1972). Developmental changes in neurochemistry during the maturation of sleep behavior. In C. D. Clemente, D. P. Purpura, & F. E. Mayer (Eds.), *Sleep and the Maturing Nervous System* (pp. 125–138). New York: Academic Press.

Holditch-Davis, D. (1990). The development of sleeping and waking states in high-risk preterm infants. *Infant Behavior and Development, 13*, 513–531.

Holditch-Davis, D., & Thoman, E. B. (1987). Behavioral states of premature infants: implications for neural and behavioral development. *Developmental Psychobiology, 20(1)*, 25–38.

Hopkins, B., & von Wulfften Palthe, T. (1987). The development of the crying state during early infancy. *Developmental Psychobiology, 20(2)*, 165–175.

Ingersoll, E. W., & Thoman, E. B. (1994). The breathing bear: effects on respiration in premature infants. *Physiology & Behavior, 56(5)*, 855–859.

Janos, O., & Papousek, H. (1977). Acquisition of appetitional and palpebral conditioned reflexes by the same infants. *Early Human Development, 1(1)*, 91–97.

Korner, A. F. (1974). The effect of the infant's states, level of arousal, sex, and ontogenetic stage on the caregiver. In M. Lewis & L. Rosenblum (Eds.), *The Effect of the Infant on its Caregiver* (pp. 105–122). John Wiley. New York.

Kronauer, R. E., Czeisler, C. A., Pilato, S. F., Moore-Ede, M. C., & Weitzman, E. D. (1982). Mathematical model of the human circadian system with two interacting oscillators. *American Physiological Society, 242(1)*, R3–R17.

Lester, B. M., & Zeskind, P. S. (1982). A biobehavioral perspective on crying in early infancy. In Fitzgerald, Lester, B. M. & Yogman (Eds.), *Theory and Research in Behavioral Pediatrics* (pp. 133–180). Vol. Plenum Press. New York

Lewis, M., & Goldberg, S. (1965). Perceptual-cognitive development in infancy: a generalized expectancy model as a function of the mother-infant interaction. *Merrill-Palmer Quarterly, 15*, 81–100.

Mahrer, A. R., Levinson, J. R., & Fine, S. (1976). Infant psychotherapy: theory, research, and practice. *Psychotherapy Theory, Research and Practice, 13*, 131–140.

Michaelis, R., Parmelee, A. H., Stern, E., & Haber, A. (1973). Activity states in premature and term infants. *Developmental Psychobiology, 6*, 209–215.

Moore, O. K. (1967). The preschool child learns to read and write. In Y. Brackbill, & G. Thompson (Eds.), *Behavior in Infancy and Early Childhood*. New York: Free Press.

Moss, H. A., & Robson, K. S. (1968). *The Role of Protest Behavior in the Development of the Mother-Infant Attachment*. American Psychological Association Conference, San Francisco.

Newson, J. (1974). Towards a theory of infant understanding. *Bulletin British Psychological Society, 27*, 251–257.

Papousek, M., Papousek, H., & Harris, B. J. (1984). The emergence of play in parent-infant interactions. In D. Görlitz & J. F. Wohlwill (Eds.), *Curiosity, Imagination, and Play. On the Development of Spontaneous Cognitive and Motivational Processes*. Hillsdale, NJ: Lawrence Erlbaum.

Prechtl, H. F. R. (1965). Problems of behavioural studies in the newborn infant. In D. S. Lehrman, R. A. Hinde, & E. Shaw (Eds.), *Advances in the Study of Behaviour* (pp. 75–96). Academic Press: New York

Prensky, A. L. (1978). Developmental disorders of the central nervous system. In S. G. Elaisson, A. L. Prensky, & W. B. J. Hardin (Eds.), *Neurological Pathophysiology* (2nd ed., pp. 3–15). New York: Oxford University Press.

Pugsley, M., Acebo, C., & Thoman, E. B. (1988). *Sleep of Preterm and Fullterm Infants From Home Monitoring*. Sixth Biennial International Conference on Infant Studies, Washington, D.C., *Infant Behavior & Development*, Special ICIS Issue.

Smotherman, W. P., & Robinson, S. R. (1987). Prenatal influences on development: behavior is not a trivial aspect of fetal life. *Developmental and Behavioral Pediatrics, 8 (3)*, 171–176.

Thoman, E. B. (1975a). Early development of sleeping behaviors in infants. In N. R. Ellis (Ed.), *Aberrant Development in Infancy: Human and Animal Studies.* (pp. 122–138). New York: John Wiley.

Thoman, E. B. (1975b). Sleep and wake behaviors in the neonates: consistencies and consequences. *Merrill-Palmer Quarterly, 21*, 295–314.

Thoman, E. B. (1981a). Affective communication as the prelude and context for language learning. In R. L. Schiefelbusch & D. Bricker (Eds.), *Early Language: Acquisition and Intervention* (pp. 181–200). Baltimore: University Park Press.

Thoman, E. B. (1981b). Early communication as the prelude to later adaptive behaviors. In M. J. Begab, H. C. Haywood, & H. Garber (Eds.), *Psychosocial Influences in Retarded Performance, Vol. II: Strategies for Improving Competence* (pp. 219–244). Baltimore: University Park Press.

Thoman, E. B. (1982). A biological perspective and a behavioral model for assessment of premature infants. In L. A. Bond & J. M. Joffe (Eds.), *Primary Prevention of Psychopathology, Vol. 6: Facilitating Infant and Early Childhood Development* (pp. 159–179). Hanover, NH: University Press of New England.

Thoman, E. B. (1985). Affects of earliest infancy: the imperative for a biological model. In E. T. McDonald & D. L. Gallagher (Eds.), *Facilitating Social-Emotional Developmental in Multiply Handicapped Children* (pp. 9–27). Philadelphia: Home of the Merciful Saviour for Crippled Children.

Thoman, E. B. (1986). Assessment of neurobehavioral stability in infants. In N. A. Krasnegor, T. I. Thompson, & D. B. Gray (Eds.), *Advances in Behavioral Pharmacology Series. Vol. 6: Developmental Behavioral Pharmacology* (pp. 79–97). Hillsdale, NJ: Lawrence Erlbaum.

Thoman, E. B. (1990). Sleeping and waking states in infants: a functional perspective. *Neuroscience and Biobehavioral Reviews, 14 (1)*, 93–107.

Thoman, E. B. (1993). Obligation and option in the premature nursery. *Developmental Review, 13*, 1–30.

Thoman, E. B., & Acebo, C. (1984). The first affections of infancy. In R. W. Bell, J. W. Elias, R. L. Greene, & J. H. Harvey (Eds.), *Interfaces in Psychology I: Developmental Psychobiology and Neuropsychology* (pp. 17–56). Lubbock: Texas Tech University Press.

Thoman, E. B., Acebo, C., & Becker, P. T. (1983). Infant crying and stability in the mother-infant relationship: a systems analysis. *Child Development, 54*, 653–659.

Thoman, E. B., Acebo, C., Dreyer, C. A., Becker, P. T., & Freese, M. P. (1979). Individuality in the interactive process. In E. B. Thoman (Ed.), *Origins of the Infant's Social Responsiveness* (pp. 305–338). Hillsdale, NJ: Lawrence Erlbaum.

Thoman, E. B., & Arnold, W. J. (1968). Effects of incubator rearing with social deprivation on maternal behavior in rats. *Journal of Comparative and Physiological Psychology, 65*, 441–446.

Thoman, E. B., & Becker, P. T. (1979). Issues in assessment and prediction for the infant born at risk. In T. Field, A. Sostek, S. Goldberg, & H. H. Shuman (Eds.), *Infants Born at Risk* (pp. 461–483). New York: Spectrum.

Thoman, E. B., Becker, P. T., & Freese, M. P. (1978). Individual patterns of mother-infant interaction. In G. P. Sacket (Ed.), *Observing Behavior, Vol. I: Theory and Applications in Mental Retardation* (pp. 95–114). Baltimore: University Park Press.

Thoman, E. B., Davis, D. H., & Denenberg, V. H. (1987). The sleeping and waking states of infants: correlations across time and person. *Physiology & Behavior, 41*, 531–537.

Thoman, E. B., Davis, D. H., Graham, S., Scholz, J. P., & Rowe, J. C. (1988). Infants at risk for Sudden Infant Death Syndrome: differential prediction for three siblings of SIDS infants. *Journal of Behavioral Medicine, 11 (6)*, 565–583.

Thoman, E. B., Denenberg, V. H., Sievel, J., Zeidner, L., & Becker, P. T. (1981). State organization in neonates: developmental inconsistency indicates risk for developmental dysfunction. *Neuropediatrics, 12*, 45–54.

Thoman, E. B., & Glazier, R. C. (1987). Computer scoring of motility patterns for states of sleep and wakefulness: human infants. *Sleep, 10(2)*, 122–129.

Thoman, E. B., & Graham, S. E. (1986). Self-regulation of stimulation by premature infants. *Pediatrics, 78(5)*, 855–860.

Thoman, E. B., Hammond, K., Affleck, G., & DeSilva, H. N. (1995). The breathing bear with premature infants: effects on sleep, respiration, and affect. *Infant Mental Health Journal, 16(3)*, 160–168.

Thoman, E. B., & Ingersoll, E. W. (1989). The human nature of the youngest humans: prematurely born babies. *Seminars in Perinatology, 13(6)*, 482–494.

Thoman, E. B., & Ingersoll, E. W. (1993). Learning in prematures. *Developmental Psychology, 29(4)*, 692–700.

Thoman, E. B., Ingersoll, E. W., & Acebo, C. (1991). Premature infants seek rhythmic stimulation, and the experience facilitates neurobehavioral development. *Journal of Development and Behavioral Pediatrics, 12*, 11–18.

Thoman, E. B., Korner, A. F., & Kraemer, H. C. (1976). Individual consistency in behavioral states in neonates. *Developmental Psychobiology, 9*, 271–283.

Thoman, E. B., Miano, V. N., & Freese, M. P. (1978). The role of respiratory instability in SIDS. *Development Medicine and Child Neurology, 19*, 748–756.

Thoman, E. B., & Pugsley, M. (1986). Stability of sleep states in infants monitored in the home. In G. V. Kondraske & C. J. Robinson (Eds.) *Eighth Annual IEEE/Engineering in Medicine and Biology Society 86CH2368–9*, 199–202.

Thoman, E. B., & Tynan, W. D. (1979). Sleep states and wakefulness in human infants: profiles from motility monitoring. *Physiology and Behavior, 23*, 519–525.

Thoman, E. B., & Whitney, M. P. (1989). Sleep states of infants monitored in the home: individual differences, developmental trends, and origins of diurnal cyclicity. *Infant Behavior and Development, 12*, 59–75.

Thoman, E. B., & Whitney, M. P. (1990). Behavioral states in infants: individual differences and individual analyses. In J. Colombo & J. W. Fagen (Eds.), *Individual Differences in Infancy: Reliability, Stability, and Prediction* (pp. 113–135). Hillsdale, NJ: Lawrence Erlbaum.

Thoman, E. B., & Zeidner, L. P. (1979). Sleep-wake states in infant rabbits: profiles from motility monitoring. *Physiology and Behavior, 22*, 1049–1054.

Tynan, W. D. (1986). Behavioral stability predicts morbidity and mortality in infants from a neonatal intensive care unit. *Infant Behavior Development, 9*, 71–79.

Valdes-Depena, M. A. (1982). *The Sudden Infant Death Syndrome: Recent Advances in Research*. Conference on Infant Apnea, Palm Springs, CA.

Weiss, P. (1969). The living system: determinism stratified. In A. Koestler & J. R. Smythies (Eds.), *Beyond Reductionism* (pp. 3–42). Boston: Beacon.

Weiss, P. (1971). The basic concept of hierarchical systems. In P. Weiss (Ed.), *Hierarchically Organized Systems in Theory and Practice*. New York: Hafner.

White, B. L. (1972). An analysis of excellent early educational practices: preliminary report. In A. Effrat (Ed.), *Interchange*. Toronto, Canada: Ontario Institute for Studies in Education.

Whitney, M. P., & Thoman, E. B. (1993). Early sleep patterns of premature infants are differentially related to later developmental disabilities. *Journal of Developmental and Behavioral Pediatrics, 14(2),* 71–80.

Winfree, A. T. (1967). Biological rhythms and the behavior of populations of coupled oscillators. *Journal of Theoretical Biology, 16,* 15–42.

Wolff, P. H. (1966). The causes, controls, and organization of behavior in the neonate. *Psychological Issues, 5(1),* 1–106.

Zeskind, P. S., & Shingler, E. A. (1991). Child abusers' perceptual responses to newborn infant cries varying in pitch. *Infant Behavior and Development, 14,* 335–347.

8

CLINICAL AND RESEARCH IMPLICATIONS FOR DEVELOPMENTAL INTERVENTIONS IN THE NEONATAL INTENSIVE CARE UNIT

ANITA MILLER SOSTEK
EDWARD GOLDSON

One of the purposes of this volume was to bring together, under one cover, the major developmental interventions that have been proposed for the very sick infant. These interventions include the individualized care of the preterm infant, kangaroo care, massage, water beds, and autonomic entrainment. Because many of these interventions remain controversial, the authors have provided theoretical rationales and experimental data to support the efficacy of each such intervention. As presented, it would seem that each intervention should stand on its own. However, this may not necessarily be the case. For example, once the infant is physiologically stable, combinations of interventions could be employed to facilitate optimal state organization and physiological stability. Individualized care could be combined with use of the water bed. As an infant becomes increasingly stable, massage could be instituted as an active intervention whereas entrainment using the Breathing Bear could be employed when the infant is alone. Finally, as an infant becomes more mature and stable and the parent more comfortable, kangaroo care could be instituted in conjunction with the other interventions, or it might be instituted shortly after birth depending on the infant's physiological and behavioral state.

Some interventions might have deleterious effects for an infant that could be monitored as its behavior and physiological state are closely observed. Although this scenario, or its variations, remains speculative, it is important to examine these interventions critically. Thus, the purpose of this overview is to summarize and integrate the information provided in this volume, to consider how these approaches can be used in a wider clinical arena, and to consider implications of these interventions for current neonatal intensive care. Finally, implications and directions for further research will be considered.

PREMATURITY AND THE NEONATAL INTENSIVE CARE UNIT

One of the most striking characteristics of the immature, preterm infant is his or her general physiological instability and, more specifically, neurological immaturity. This phenomenon has been amply described in the literature (Avery, Fletcher, & McDonald, 1994) and has been of considerable concern to medical caretakers, parents, and researchers alike. An infant's immaturity is reflected in the instability of vital signs; a lack of coordination in the ability to suck, swallow, and breath at the same time until about 32 weeks (Prechtl et al., 1979); an inability to modulate physiologic responses to stress (Gorski, 1983; Gorski et al., 1983); and behavioral disorganization as reflected in disorganized state control and poor ability to participate in social interactions. Thus, much of what happens in the neonatal intensive care unit (NICU) serves to maintain an infant, from a physiological viewpoint, until it is capable of sustaining itself independently. This is the reason for the use of the ventilator; surfactant; nitric oxide; parenteral, gavage, or gastrostomy feeds; the incubator, and all of the other medical interventions and supports employed in the care of a very small baby.

When one considers the role of developmental interventions, a somewhat different, but not mutually exclusive, perspective is taken. A review of the chapters included in this volume, reveals that all of the suggested interventions seek, using one or another technique or approach, to ameliorate not only physiological instability but also behavioral disorganization. Frequently, the physiological and behavioral capacities of the premature infant are viewed separately in the NICU and so the focus of interventions employed differs. That is to say, energy may be expended in sustaining the infant from a pulmonary viewpoint, without taking into serious consideration the effect of these interventions on other organ systems and the need to gauge the infant's responses, both physiological and behavioral, outside of the pulmonary domain.

The thrust of this volume, and the message it seeks to convey, is that behavior and physiology are not separate entities. On the contrary, they are intimately linked and influence each other in profound ways. The behaviorally organized infant is a reflection of its intact, functioning central nervous system (CNS). The functioning of the CNS, setting aside anatomic abnormalities, depends on and reflects the stability of the cardiopulmonary, renal, and hematopoietic systems. Therefore, an intervention in one system is bound to have an effect on the other systems. Thus, among the questions raised in the care of the premature infant is what kind of nonmedical, developmental interventions can be employed to enhance the fragile infant's physiological stability and behavioral organization. Furthermore, what measures can be employed to assess the effects, both positive and negative, of these interventions on the infant?

Although it has been argued that all systems are linked, it can also be argued that there is a hierarchy of supports necessary for physiological systems. The first priority, of course, is to have a live infant! Next, one could argue that the infant needs some degree of physiological stability before it can be manipulated. Once this has been accomplished, other needs can be addressed. It is also important to take into consideration the environment in which the infant finds him or herself. Goldson (Chapter 1; this volume; 1992) and others (Glass, 1994; Graven et al., 1992) have described the NICU as an intrusive, noncontingent, and potentially overstimulating environment that at the same time, lacks modulated stimulation. The NICU tends to function and respond to its own rhythms rather than to the rhythms and cues of the infant. In contrast to both the home environment and the intrauterine environment, it is extremely noisy and bright, with minimal social interaction and little diurnal patterning. Physical interventions are performed repeatedly, often with scant attention to an infant's physiological and behavioral state. Models of developmental intervention need to recognize the primary aims of the NICU. At the same time, they need to examine the elements that can be altered in the NICU organizational, sensory, and social domains to achieve responsivity to an infant's cues and thus support and facilitate physiological and behavioral organization.

MODELS OF INTERVENTION

Ramey (chapter 3, this volume) presents a theoretical framework for conceptualizing risk and intervention during and after the NICU hospitalization. Risk is a probabilistic notion and includes both reproductive and caretaking casualty (Knobloch & Pasamanick, 1966; Sameroff & Chandler, 1975). Risk diminishes when an infant comes from a resourceful family that can use the supports provided from within as well as from the wider community. Risk changes at different developmental points, and the nature of appropriate interventions changes accordingly. In the NICU, the majority of the interventions are physical, but the foundation also needs to be laid for developmental and familial interventions. Developmental interventions in the NICU have been based on the following features: (1) theories of normalizing and humanizing, (2) adding supplemental stimulation in order to compensate for the presumed sensory deprivation, and (3) compensating for the loss of the intrauterine environment. Ramey argues that, regardless of theoretical orientation, the efficacy of an intervention depends on an infant's physiological, behavioral and neuromaturational status, the physical environment, and the nature of the caregiver. Family intervention also depends, in part, on caregivers' perceptions of the infant. The perception of fragility, for example, may lead to overprotection and unnecessary limitations on social and locomotor opportunities. The preparation that the NICU staff can provide a family should include a realistic portrayal of an infant's abilities and limitations, as well as ongoing methods for assessing the baby's receptivity and stress.

Ramey's emphasis on the poor fit between the NICU environment and an infant's needs and abilities supports the individualized approach to care described by Als (Chapter 2, this volume). Although risk must be seen in the context of the larger environment of the infant, the effects on the infant of the timing, breadth, and intensity of medical interventions in the NICU, along with various developmental interventions, remain unknown. At the most basic level, the work of Als addresses the initial attempts to handle a fragile infant in the most nonintrusive, yet developmentally appropriate, manner while he or she is cared for in a generally intensive, noncontingent setting. Als presents a model of NICU care that emphasizes whatever regulation and organization is possible within the context of medical necessity. She maintains that infants participate actively in their own care and help shape their own development. Systematic observations of infants' behavior, state regulation, signs of stress, and receptivity are emphasized. Critically important is the behavioral state regulation of the infants. Physical caregiving must be linked to behavioral state in order to minimize excess energy expenditure and allow for maximum brain growth. Behavior needs to be systematically observed to provide cues for the timing and intensity of physical, social, and feeding interventions. Sensory stimulation in all modalities is modulated and organized around periods of alertness. Physical positioning of the infant should promote flexion and midline positioning, and treatments are clustered to avoid frequent disturbance to an infant and are offered only if actually necessary. The NICU caregivers work in primary care teams so that the staff knows each infant well. Finally, and most important, the parents are encouraged to assume an active role in the NICU and provide skin-to-skin contact whenever possible as a means of physiologically stabilizing and soothing the infant.

Als compares preterm groups who received or did not receive contingent, sensitive care with one another as well as with a full-term group. The benefits of the intervention in the nursery include less need for ventilatory support, less tone during gavage feedings, greater weight gain, shorter hospitalization time, and improved short-term developmental outcome. At 9 months, the infants in the contingent care group had higher mental developmental scores, performed better on problem-solving tasks using the kangaroo box, and generally appeared more organized and well modulated (Als et al., 1994). The authors speculate that the intervention was effective either by promoting brain development or by reducing episodes of hypoxia because the infants were less stressed.

SPECIFIC INTERVENTIONS

Anderson (Chapter 6, this volume) advocates the expanded use of skin-to-skin contact between the infant and the mother (or father) in the form of kangaroo care. She has taken an approach to caring for healthy and sick infants that has been well accepted in many countries in the past. Even for the sickest babies, kangaroo care has been found to be safe for the infant and beneficial to the caretaker. In describing her approach, Anderson, like Als, advocates that an infant be closely monitored, that its cues be read and correctly interpreted, and that it be given the opportunity to participate in the caretaking process and to be protected from possible adverse effects. Anderson presents work by herself and others that demonstrates that kangaroo care can be used with mature infants, stable infants on ventilators, and very immature infants who have difficulty with thermal control.

The major focus of much of the current work concerning kangaroo care has been to establish its safety. However, there is compelling evidence that this intervention has a positive physiological effect on the infant in the form of decreased apnea, better temperature control, less crying and irritability, and enhanced state organization. It has been shown to enhance mother's milk production and to help in establishing and sustaining a more meaningful relationship between a parent and child. By its nature, it provides a transition from illness to health and also helps an infant to establish its own personhood. It also combines well with other developmental interventions that can also be used to enhance neurobehavioral maturation and organization.

Korner (Chapter 5, this volume) addresses a somewhat different approach to the premature infants; she presents the rationale, method, and effect of a form of vestibular, or movement, stimulation on the premature infant. The intervention is based on the assumption that a premature infant is deprived of stimulation and that compensatory forms of stimulation, similar to those available *in utero*, will optimize its functioning, although it is not actually a replication of the intrauterine experience. It was also hoped that this stimulation would protect an infant's skin and might reduce the incidence of the oddly shaped, oblong heads frequently encountered in very immature infants. Drawing on the theoretical construct and evidence from primate and nonprimate studies, Korner decided to use the oscillating water bed for this compensatory movement stimulation.

To evaluate the effect of this intervention, a series of studies first demonstrated that water beds were safe for most infants. Moreover, infants placed on the beds had much less apnea and irritability, particularly when the oscillating bed was used. An exception to these findings lay in unstable infants with endocrine or cardiopulmonary disturbances; they deteriorated under these conditions. Other studies found that, with the use of the oscillating water bed, infants demonstrated more mature motor behavior along with decreased apnea. Infants also were more visually alert, attended better, and had better pursuit of inanimate and animate auditory and visual stimuli. In short, infants with uncomplicated apnea exposed to this form of compensatory vestibular stimuli were better organized than controls. Based on these data, this developmental intervention can be used safely even with extremely premature infants to optimize their state control, physiologic stability, and interactive capacities. Under controlled monitored conditions, this intervention could also be included in the individualized care plan proposed by Als, thereby extending the small infant's range of positive, contingent experiences.

The water bed is an intervention that can be used quite early in an infant's course as long as he or she can tolerate it. On the other hand, the intervention proposed by Thoman (Chapter 7, this volume) for more mature premature infants taps into an infant's emerging capabilities for self-regulation. Thoman and her colleagues postulated that an infant would prefer and respond to an object that provided it with a rhythmic stimulus and that he or she had the capability of making contact with this object. They developed a breathing toy bear for this purpose. They further hypothesized that such an experience would facilitate the maturation of neurodevelopmental processes. Thoman was able to demonstrate that premature infants at 32 to 34 weeks postconceptual age were able to organize their motor movements such that they approached and maintained contact with the Breathing Bear. Moreover, the infant was found to be capable of entrainment and of learning from exposure to this rhythmic stimulus. The infants exposed to the Breathing Bear seemed to have more advanced neurobehavioral development as evidenced by greater regularity of quiet sleep (QS) and decreased frequency of arousal movements in QS. Finally, more positive affect was associated with exposure to the Breathing Bear, expressed by less crying, more smiling, and better organization of sleep/wake cycles. The most significant aspect of these results is that those infants exposed to the Breathing Bear demonstrated a greater capacity for self-regulation, which allows them to become more active participants in their environment. Consequently, their neurobehavioral competence is enhanced as well as their role as social partners.

The infants exposed to the Breathing Bear "chose" to establish and maintain contact with the object providing them with a positive, rhythmic stimulus. These studies suggest that neurobehavioral development can be facilitated in the intact premature infant who is provided with an opportunity to control his or her environment. Questions remain as to whether this also applies to the very premature infant or the damaged infant and whether this intervention ameliorates the effects of CNS injury or prolonged illness.

In Chapter 4, Field, like Anderson, incorporates cross-cultural practices into neonatal care by adopting massage for infants at risk. Massage therapy extends the emphasis on early stimulation that started in the 1970s and demonstrates that relatively vigorous tactile stimulation can be applied to preterm infants during their "grower" period when they are out of medical crisis and primarily gaining weight. The massage includes stroking and kinesthetic stimulation. In the studies described, massaged infants gained weight more rapidly; were more awake and responsive; performed better on behavioral assessments of habituation, orientation, motor activity, and state regulation; and went home earlier than nonmassaged infants. In addition to growing preterms, massage is beneficial for special infants at risk, such as those exposed to cocaine or HIV. Field and her colleagues have explored the physiological, hormonal, and digestive effects of massage in rats (Schanberg & Field, 1988). Although the mechanisms by which massage is effective are not well understood, possible explanations include alterations in the secretion of food absorption hormones and reduction in stress. Schanberg and Field also found that benefits of providing massage can extend to an infant's caregivers, who can gain a feeling of efficacy and take a more active role in its care. Benefits have been demonstrated in mothers with depression, as well as in grandparent volunteers. Like kangaroo care, water beds, and the Breathing Bear, massage is a low-technology approach to the care of infants at risk that appears to have positive economic, physical, and emotional effects.

CLINICAL IMPLICATIONS

The issues that emerge from the studies presented in this volume raise the need to consider additional approaches to the management of the very small infant.

There is no question that the most pressing task for the staff of the NICU is to maintain life. However, there may be other, nonmedical, interventions that can facilitate this task and also contribute to neurobehavioral organization and development. The interventions described in this volume attest first to the fact that alterations or additions to medical care unharmful to the infant can be made. Moreover, there is strong evidence that, when monitored closely, these interventions can have a positive effect not only on the infant but also on the staff and family.

A second issue that emerges is the need to change the current perception of the sick infant as a passive organism. All of the interventions described amply demonstrate that an infant has the capacity to be an active participant in his or her environment and care. Moreover, the approaches described demonstrate that this capacity can be enhanced using appropriate interventions utilized in response to an infant's cues. This then leads to the third issue, the need to endow the tiny infant with "personhood." Als's approach speaks to this challenge as the efficacy of an intervention depends on the caretakers' ability to respond to an infant's physiologic and behavioral cues. Furthermore, the close interaction involved in kangaroo care and the active participation of an infant in responding to the breathing bear help to emphasize the individuality of the infant and his or her ability to respond to the physical and social environment. This individuality and responsivity help involve the caregivers and offer them a more positive experience when engaging in caregiving activities.

The volume emphasizes multimodal interventions including modulated and organized experiences in the vestibular, postural, visual, tactile, and auditory domains. A blend of approaches directed by an infant's cues is probably the best way to optimize the efficacy of developmental interventions. These approaches must allow an infant to be an active participant whose activity and responses are observed to a great enough extent that they can help direct the caregivers to organize the infant's care. Furthermore, inclusion of parents and other nonmedical caregivers benefits both the infants and the adults involved with it.

From a theoretical viewpoint, these interventions appear to make sense. But there are pressing questions that need to be answered if these interventions are to be widely used as the accepted standard of care. Above all, they should cause no harm—*primum non nocere*. Since this seems to be the case, the question is raised as to whether they should be widely used and who should be providing the care. What is the cost to implement these interventions and are there savings in the long run? As compared to the current standard of care, do they truly make a positive difference, and do they positively affect long-term outcome for this very high-risk population of infants?

The work of Als has generated considerable controversy; it is the most involved of the interventions, implemented very shortly after birth. Furthermore, it requires intensive training of caretakers and considerable expertise and ongoing assessment. Als (Chapter 2, this volume; Als et al., 1995) has demonstrated that this intervention reduces common serious morbidities in ventilated, very low birthweight infants. Additionally, they had more rapid weight gain, im-

proved short-term neurodevelopmental outcome, shorter hospital stays, and reduced hospital bills. The other interventions—oscillating water beds, massage,
kangaroo care and the Breathing Bear—have also been shown to be safe, to
enhance weight gain, to increase neurobehavioral organization, to reduce hospital stays, and to facilitate the caregiver-infant relationship. It appears that the
relatively small investment in individualized, contingent care has benefited the
infant, the hospital caretakers, and the parents as it reduces the hospital cost.
One of the questions that needs to asked is whether hospitals are willing to take
the time and make the effort to implement these additions to current care. Before
this will occur, the interventions must be replicated at different sites to convince
neonatologists and administrators that these are cost-effective, safe, efficacious
interventions both in the short term and over the long term.

RESEARCH ISSUES

As alluded to previously, there still is a great need to replicate these interventions
in other settings and to determine that, in other hands, they can be effectively
employed. This has taken place with the individualized care plan proposed by
Als and kangaroo care proposed by Anderson. However, even more basic research questions emerge. What is the mechanism by which these interventions
work? Each of the authors has started to address this question, but there is much
work still to be done.

A question of considerable basic science and clinical interest with respect to
Als's work is whether one can break down the entire intervention into its individual components. If so, which of the components are the most efficacious and
how do they all fit together? Going a step further, do different interventions
introduced simultaneously or sequentially affect the infant? What are the mechanisms by which these individual interventions applied in concert cause an effect? What is the nature and magnitude of the effect? Field and her coworkers
have started this work by suggesting that massage affects the secretion of gastric
hormones, which enhances absorption and utilization of nutrients, which, in
turn, enhances weight gain and neurodevelopmental stability, thereby allowing
for shorter hospital stays. This is a beginning, but again, much work remains.
Individualized developmental care needs to be tried and tested for its efficacy,
with short-term and long-term neurodevelopmental outcome as the basis for the
evaluation (Merenstein, 1994).

If one allows that all of the developmental interventions described in this
volume are efficacious in enhancing physiologic stability and neurodevelopmental organization, still these questions remain: when should they be introduced,
in what sequence should they be introduced, and are they all necessary to accomplish the desired effect. To date, all of these interventions appear to have
been used in isolation. Are there synergistic effects? How does one measure the
effect of multimodal interventions? What new assessment strategies are required
to determine efficacy to convince the basic scientist as well as the clinician? In
the past, different strategies have been used to evaluate early intervention pro-

grams. Can these be used to assess the effect of these neonatal interventions? Should different outcome models be used that move away from looking at standardized test scores and use functional assessments (Saigal et al., 1990)? This area certainly needs much research and lends itself to collaboration between clinicians and basic scientists.

Of considerable interest is the fact that some of the interventions appear to have been utilized primarily for more stable premature infants, whereas others have been used on extremely sick, fragile babies. Are the interventions necessarily limited to these different groups of infants? For example, can the former interventions be used for sicker infants safely and do they have positive effects? Similarly, are the more extensive interventions necessary, or even effective, for the more stable infant? Does a combination of interventions have the greatest effect? How do each of these approaches compare to the more traditional care currently employed? Answers are considerably important for clinical practice, particularly when financial and personnel resources are becoming increasingly limited.

Finally, there are short-term neurodevelopmental benefits following all of the interventions. Are these gains sustained over the long term and what are the appropriate outcome measures to assess their efficacy? Are other interventions required to sustain these initial positive effects? Demonstrating both short-term and long-term gains associated with these interventions would provide a powerful argument for their inclusion in the current care of sick and immature infants. Recent studies reveal that 10% of infants with birthweights < 1,500 g have significant neurologic abnormalities and that, of the remaining "normal" children tested at school age, some 60% have significant learning or behavioral difficulties (Goldson, 1996b). This is even more so the case for the *micropremie*, an infant with birthweights < 800 g (Goldson, 1996b). It is critical to evaluate the potential of the interventions described in this book to lead to better outcomes for these high-risk infants.

SUMMARY

We have attempted in this chapter to review a number of developmental interventions proposed for inclusion in the care of the very sick infant. We described the environment of the NICU and then discussed a model for early intervention that lead to a discussion of the individual interventions. The clinical implications of interventions were identified and suggestions for further research proposed. Certainly many more questions can be raised and these, one hopes, will emerge with more research. It is clear that these interventions are safe, efficacious at least in the short term, and financially advantageous. It is now for the reader to determine whether and how they can be implemented into current care of the newborn. If we have stimulated our readers to consider incorporating these interventions in the care of the sick infant, our mission in editing this book and writing this critique has been accomplished.

REFERENCES

Als, H., Lawhon, G., Duffy, F. H., McAnulty, G. B., Gibes-Grossman, R., & Blickman, J. G. (1994). Individualized developmental care for the very low-birth-weight preterm infant. *Journal of the American Medical Association, 272*, 853–858.

Avery, G. B., Fletcher, M. A., & McDonald, M. G. (1994). *Neonatal Pathophysiology and Management of the Newborn* (4th ed.). Philadelphia: J. B. Lippincott.

Glass, P. (1994). The vulnerable neonate and the neonatal intensive care environment. In G. B. Avery, M. A. Fletcher, & M. G. McDonald (Eds.), *Neonatal Pathophysiology and Management of the Newborn* (4th ed., pp. 71–91). Philadelphia: J. B. Lippincott.

Goldson, E. (1992). Neonatal intensive care unit: premature infants and parents. *Infants and Young Children, 4*, 4 31–42.

Goldson, E. (1996a). The micropremie: infants with birthweight < 800 grams. *Inf. Young Children.*

Goldson, E. (1996b). Follow-up of very low birth weight infants: neurodevelopmental and educational sequelae. In M. L. Wolraich (Ed.), *The Practical Assessment and Management of Children with Disorders of Development and Learning* (2nd ed). Chicago: Mosby-Year Book.

Gorski, P. A. (1983). Premature infant behavioral and physiologic responses to caregiving interventions in the intensive care nursery. In J. D. Call, E. Galenson, & R. L. Tyson (Eds.), *Frontiers in Infant Psychiatry* (pp. 256–263). New York: Basic Books.

Gorski, P. A., Hole, W. T., Leonard, C. H., & Martin, J. A. (1983). Direct computer recording of premature infants and nursery care. *Pediatrics, 72*, 198–202.

Graven, S. N., Bowen, F. W., Brooten, D., Eaton, A., et al. (1992). The high risk infant environment, Part I. The role of the neonatal intensive care unit in the outcome of high-risk infants. *Journal of Perinatology, 12*, 164–172.

Knobloch, H., & Pasamanick, B. (1966). Prospective studies on the epidemiology of reproductive casualty: methods, findings, and some implications. *Merrill-Palmer Quarterly, 12*, 27–36.

Merenstein, G. B. (1994). Individualized developmental care: an emerging new standard for neonatal intensive care units? *Journal of the American Medical 272*, 890–891.

Prechtl, H. F. R., Fargel, J. W., Weinmann, H. M., & Bakker, H. H. (1979). Posture, motility and respiration in low-risk preterm infants. *Developmental Medicine and Child Neurology, 21*, 3–27.

Saigal, S., Szatmari, P., Rosenbaum, P., Campbell, D., & King, S. (1990). Intellectual and functional status at school entry of children who weighed 1,000 grams or less at birth: regional perspective of birth in the 1980's. *The Journal of Pediatrics,116*, 409–416.

Sameroff, A. J., & Chandler, M. (1975). Reproductive risk and the continuum of caretaking casualty. In F. D. Horowitz, E. M. Hetherington, S. Scarr-Salapatek, & G. Siegel (Eds.), *Review of Child Development Research* (Vol. 4, pp. 187–243). Chicago: University of Chicago Press.

Schanberg, S., & Field, T. (1988). Maternal deprivation and supplemental stimulation. In T. Field, P. McCabe, & N. Schneiderman (Eds.), *Stress and Coping Across Development.* Hillsdale, NJ: Lawrence Erlbaum.

Index

Page numbers followed by f and t indicate figures and tables, respectively.